Journal of Health Politics, Policy and Law

Editor Jonathan Oberlander, University of North Carolina at Chapel Hill

Associate Editors Nicholas Bagley, University of Michigan; Sarah E. Gollust, University of Minnesota; Helen Levy, University of Michigan; Elizabeth Rigby, George Washington University

Book Review Editor Miriam J. Laugesen, Columbia University

Special Section Editors Beneath the Surface: Joseph White, Case Western Reserve University; Tracking Health Reform: Heather Howard, Princeton University, and Frank J. Thompson, Rutgers University

Social Media Editor Harold A. Pollack, University of Chicago

Managing Editor Jed P. Cohen

Former Editors Ralph A. Straetz, New York University; Theodore R. Marmor, Yale University; Lawrence D. Brown, Columbia University; James A. Morone, Brown University; Mark A. Peterson, University of California, Los Angeles; Mark Schlesinger, Yale University; Michael S. Sparer, Columbia University; Colleen M. Grogan, University of Chicago; Eric M. Patashnik, Brown University

Volume 46, Number 5, October 2021
Published by Duke University Press

Contents

Introduction: Investigating Dimensions of Pandemic Inequity Requires a Multidisciplinary Approach

Sarah E. Gollust
University of Minnesota

Julia Lynch
University of Pennsylvania

When the coronavirus emerged in the United States in early 2020, reassuring early platitudes suggested that "we are all in this together" and "COVID-19 is an equal opportunity killer" (see, e.g., Blow 2020; Reuters 2020). These platitudes quickly became exposed as such, however, as evidence demonstrating the unequal reach and consequences of the pandemic accumulated. Data on the epidemiologic impact—combined with the everyday experiences of the most affected groups in the United States—continue to reinforce the reality that this pandemic is inequitable in almost every imaginable dimension. According to March 2021 data from the Color of Coronavirus project, the highest overall rates of death are among Indigenous Americans (256 deaths per 100,000), followed by Black Americans (180 deaths per 100,000); once accounting for age, Pacific Islanders and Latinos have the highest mortality rates (APM 2021). Coronavirus-related concern is also unequally distributed by race, with only 17% of white respondents to a Pew survey in late 2020 saying they were very concerned about getting COVID-19, while 37% of Hispanic and 36% of Black respondents reported the same (Pew 2020). Furthermore, 71% of Black respondents in the same poll reported they knew someone who had been hospitalized or died as a result of COVID-19, compared to 49% of white respondents (Pew 2020). Higher viral exposure through high-risk workplaces (e.g., meatpacking), living in crowded housing conditions (including long-term care and carceral settings), and inability to work from home—combined with heightened vulnerability to more serious illness because of chronic conditions borne from compounded risks of structural

Journal of Health Politics, Policy and Law, Vol. 46, No. 5, October 2021
DOI 10.1215/03616878-9155949   © 2021 by Duke University Press

racism—underscores the fundamental contribution of social and economic conditions at both the individual and community levels (Bailey and Moon 2020; Karmaker, Lantz, and Tipirneni 2021; Rollston and Galea 2020).

While these descriptive data confirm the highly unequal impact of the pandemic, a comprehensive understanding of how these inequities came to be requires a multidisciplinary approach. It is necessary to not only engage with the epidemiological issues of disease distribution but also examine the politics and policy that contribute to inequities and that could alternatively be mobilized to promote health equity. The six studies in this special issue of the *Journal of Health Politics, Policy and Law* do just that. Each article engages with the politics of inequality, demonstrating how inequality in the incidence and impact of COVID-19 was built on fundamentally unequal social, economic, and political structures in the United States and reproduced during the course of the pandemic in 2020. Using the lenses of law, political science, disability rights, and health policy, the authors contribute new insights into the politics at the center of pandemic inequality.

In the first article of this special issue, Sarah Rosenbaum, Morgan Handley, Rebecca Morris, and Maria Casoni present a case study of four ostensibly race-neutral health care policy decisions made by the Trump administration during the COVID-19 pandemic. They demonstrate that each of these policy choices exacerbated racial inequality and perpetuated structural racism. As a remedy for the future, they argue that equity must be at the center of health policy making—what they describe as an "equity-mindful" approach—which would incorporate a formal health equity assessment into the policy-making process. They suggest that such a policy-making strategy is consistent with US civil rights law, and alongside a fuller retrospective analysis of how policies in 2020 contributed to pandemic inequality, constitutes critical steps toward ameliorating structural inequities.

Consistent with Rosenbaum and colleagues' call for deeper retrospective policy evaluation, Colleen M. Grogan, Michael K. Gusmano, and Yu-An Lin analyze one of the four case studies that the previous piece highlighted, the distribution of CARES Act provider relief funds to hospitals. They evaluate the distributional schemes that the US Department of Health and Human Services applied based on two key metrics: percent of outpatient revenue (measuring those hospitals likely to suffer most from revenue losses during the early phase of COVID-19) and days of cash on hand (measuring financial vulnerability of the hospital). Based on this analysis, they conclude that the CARES Act funds enriched hospitals that were already better resourced pre-pandemic. Their article situates the CARES

Act policy response within the already bifurcated structure of the American hospital system, providing a useful narrative history of how reliance on private capital contributed to hospital stratification into "haves" and "have-nots" long before the pandemic's arrival in the United States in 2020.

While the CARES Act comprises a set of policies developed with the principal objective of providing relief from COVID-19–related burdens (on hospitals, other businesses, and the general public), Michael W. Sances and Andrea Louise Campbell's study examines whether and how existing (i.e., pre-COVID) state-level policies buffered the impact of COVID-19 on mental health. Continuing the theme established in Rosenbaum and colleagues' article, Sances and Campbell apply a structural racism lens to examine the racialized impacts of the pandemic and how existing inequalities in availability of safety-net policies (including unemployment benefits, paid sick leave, and Medicaid expansion) reinforced COVID-19–related inequality. The authors find significant consequences of the pandemic on mental health, with heightened mental distress among people of color. They further demonstrate that the effects of losing employment on mental health was offset by living in a state with a more generous safety net, illuminating the deleterious consequences of the differences in generosity across state contexts.

The next two articles offer deeper dives into two critically important—and often neglected in studies of health equity—populations: people with disabilities, and those living in carceral settings. Ari Ne'eman, Michael Ashley Stein, Zackary D. Berger, and Doron Dorfman conduct an analysis of change over time in state crisis standard of care (CSC) policies, policies that establish guidelines for triage of scarce resources. They first present a normative analysis about a set of five allocation criteria within CSC plans, suggesting which criteria promote disability rights and which are legally problematic according to disability rights law. Then they apply a rubric to code 58 CSC policies from 35 states to produce an index score reflecting degree of alignment with disability rights policy preferences. They find evidence that revisions to CSC policies over time increasingly align with disability rights and thus may reflect the influence of disability activism in public policy making. Their study presents questions for future inquiry about how the process of influence around bioethics issues happens in policy making.

Matthew G. T. Denney and Ramon Garibaldo Valdez examine the impact of COVID-19 within prisons, jails, and migrant detention centers. They first document how compounded racial vulnerability and specific policy choices contributed to the spread of COVID-19 in carceral institutions. They next ask how the general public would respond if they knew about the racial inequalities and poor health conditions within these facilities, using a survey-based experiment. While their results generally depict a public uninterested in the plight of people in these institutions, they suggest that providing information about racial disparities may lead to increased public support for decarceration.

In the final article of this special issue, Katherine Carman, Anita Chandra, Carolyn Miller, Christopher Nelson, and Jhacova Williams present a less optimistic view about the potential of public awareness of racial disparities to translate into meaningful change in policy support. They leverage panel data from 2018 and 2020 to examine changes in awareness of health inequity over time. Despite high attention among public health professionals and at least some mass media outlets to the types of inequities embodied by COVID-19, Carman and colleagues' article suggests that these ideas have not been disseminated into the general public in ways that could meaningfully shift their understanding of health inequity. While 60% of respondents to their summer 2020 survey believed (correctly) that people of color face more health impacts of COVID-19 than whites, these views were more common among respondents of color than white respondents, and among those who acknowledged in 2018 that people of color faced health care inequities. The authors suggest that this finding signifies that beliefs about health inequities are unlikely to shift in a major way in response to information from news reporting, for instance, about the relationship between structural racism and health outcomes—whether COVID-19 or other health conditions. However, the authors do observe a significant shift in the share of the public that perceives that the government has an obligation to ensure access to health care, suggesting some broad public recognition that the government has a role in reducing health inequities, even if not necessarily framed with that specific objective.

Taken together, the articles in this special issue are a powerful argument for the importance of multidisciplinary analysis of health politics, policy, and law for understanding health equity. High-quality epidemiologic and demographic approaches to health equity are essential for revealing the inequalities in exposures, susceptibilities, and outcomes generated by COVID-19. Indeed, surveillance data in 2021 demonstrate striking inequities in vaccination rates by race, with Black and Hispanic people receiving lower shares of vaccinations compared to their share of the population (Ndugga et al. 2021). But an understanding of the upstream political, policy, and legal contexts that have shaped these and other population health outcomes is equally important, especially if we want to identify levers for change that operate at the collective or structural level.

■ ■ ■

Sarah E. Gollust is an associate professor of health policy and management at the University of Minnesota and is a senior advisor of the Robert Wood Johnson Foundation's Interdisciplinary Research Leaders program. Her research examines the influence of the media and public opinion in the health policy process, the dissemination of research into policy making, and the politics of health policy. Her research has been funded by the National Institutes of Health, the Robert Wood Johnson Foundation, the Russell Sage Foundation, and the American Cancer Society. sgollust@umn.edu

Julia Lynch is a professor of political science at the University of Pennsylvania. Her research focuses on the politics of inequality and social policy in rich democracies. She has special interests in comparative health policy, the politics of public health, and aging politics and policy. Her recent books are *Regimes of Inequality: The Political Economy of Health and Wealth* (2020) and *The Unequal Pandemic: Covid-19 and Health Inequalities* (2021). jflynch@sas.upenn.edu

References

APM Research Lab. 2021. "The Color of Coronavirus: COVID-19 Deaths by Race and Ethnicity in the US." March 5. www.apmresearchlab.org/covid/deaths-by-race.

Bailey, Zinzi, and J. Robin Moon. 2020. "Racism and the Political Economy of COVID-19: Will We Continue to Resurrect the Past?" *Journal of Health Politics, Policy and Law* 45, no. 6: 937–50.

Blow, Charles M. 2020. "Social Distancing Is a Privilege." *New York Times*, April 5. nytimes.com/2020/04/05/opinion/coronavirus-social-distancing.html.

Karmakar, Monita, Paula M. Lantz, and Renuka Tipirneni. 2021. "Association of Social and Demographic Factors with COVID-19 Incidence and Death Rates in the US." *JAMA Network Open* 4, no. 1: e2036462. doi.org/10.1001/jamanetworkopen.2020.36462.

Ndugga, Nambi, Olivia Pham, Latoya Hill, Samantha Artiga, and Salem Mengistu. 2021. "Latest Data on COVID-19 Vaccinations Race/Ethnicity." Kaiser Family Foundation, March 3. www.kff.org/coronavirus-covid-19/issue-brief/latest-data-on-covid-19-vaccinations-race-ethnicity/.

Pew Research Center. 2020. "Intent to Get a COVID-19 Vaccine Rises to 60% as Confidence in Research and Development Process Increases." December 3. www.pewresearch.org/science/2020/12/03/intent-to-get-a-covid-19-vaccine-rises-to-60-as-confidence-in-research-and-development-process-increases/.

Reuters. 2020. "'We're All in This Together': Coronavirus Task Force Addresses Nation." *New York Times*, June 26. www.nytimes.com/video/us/politics/100000007211515/coronavirus-task-force-press-conference.html.

Rollston, Rebekah, and Sandro Galea. 2020. "COVID-19 and the Social Determinants of Health." *American Journal of Health Promotion* 34, no. 6: 687–89.

How the Trump Administration's Pandemic Health Care Response Failed Racial Health Equity: Case Studies of Structural Racism and a Call for Equity Mindfulness in Federal Health Policy Making

Sara Rosenbaum
Morgan Handley
Rebecca Morris
Maria Casoni
George Washington University

Abstract

Context: The racial health equity implications of the Trump administration's response to the COVID-19 pandemic.

Methods: We focus on four key health care policy decisions made by the administration in response to the public health emergency: rejecting a special Marketplace enrollment period, failing to use its full powers to enhance state Medicaid emergency options, refusing to suspend the public charge rule, and failing to target provider relief funds to providers serving the uninsured.

Findings: In each case, the administration's policy choices intensified, rather than mitigated, racial health inequality. Its choices had a disproportionate adverse impact on minority populations and patients who are more likely to depend on public programs, be poor, experience pandemic-related job loss, lack insurance, rely on health care safety net providers, and be exposed to public charge sanctions.

Conclusions: Ending structural racism in health care and promoting racial health care equity demands an equity-mindful approach to the pursuit of policies that enhance—rather than undermine—health care accessibility and effectiveness and resources for the poorest communities and the providers that serve them.

Keywords COVID-19, pandemic, Trump administration, civil rights, structural racism

That the COVID-19 pandemic would hit people and communities of color with particular force was entirely predictable. As with past pandemics (Oppenheim and Yamey 2017), COVID-19 thrives on people who experience high poverty, cramped living arrangements, unsafe residential care, elevated daily health risks, high-exposure jobs, excessive underlying health problems, reduced access to health insurance and health care, and an

Journal of Health Politics, Policy and Law, Vol. 46, No. 5, October 2021
DOI 10.1215/03616878-9155963   © 2021 by Duke University Press

inadequate public health system. Minority Americans disproportionately experience all of these risks (Oppel et al. 2020), and concentrated poverty means that these risks exist on a community-wide basis.

COVID-19 has laid bare the inequality that undergirds today's health care landscape. As David Blumenthal and colleagues (2020) point out, the novel coronavirus has done much to "reveal and compound deep underlying problems in the health care system of the United States." Among these problems are extensive racial disparities that are a manifestation of structural racism, that is, the pattern of systematic and mutually reinforcing policies that both generate and lock in racial inequity (Berkowitz et al. 2020; Egede and Walker 2020; Figueroa et al. 2020; Matthew 2015; Michener 2019; Selden and Berdahl 2020).

The problem of racism in health care in the United States has been extensively documented (Byrd and Clayton 2001; IOM 2003), and the search for solutions is not new. Ending racial inequality in health care was a central, underlying consideration in the enactment of Title VI of the 1964 Civil Rights Act (Smith 1999), which bars federally assisted entities from engaging in both intentional and de facto discrimination. By targeting both intentional acts and seemingly neutral policies with racially disproportionate effects, Title VI effectively anticipated the structural racism framework that drives the health equity discourse today.

More recently, the focus on equity has expanded beyond the conduct of recipients of federal funding to include the federal policy making process itself. Evidence of this emerging embrace of equity as a core element of federal health policy making can be seen in President Biden's executive orders, specifically, an order establishing a COVID-19 Health Equity Task Force to make recommendations regarding a broadly equitable approach to agency pandemic policy making, including funding disbursement, outreach, and communication (Biden 2021). Further evidence of a focus on equity and health policy making also can be seen in a comprehensive report issued by the US House of Representatives Ways and Means Committee (2021) focusing on equity and legislative policy.

Ending structural racism in federal health policy making begins with an effort to call out policy actions and choices that feed the problem; only then can policy makers confront the phenomenon and seek fairer and just solutions. The need to confront discriminatory federal policies is true for all forms of discrimination, whether based on race and national origin, disability, sex, or other prohibited classification, and the need for equity mindfulness is equally applicable. Here, however, we focus on the problem of racial inequity in health and health care.

The choices made by the Trump administration underscore the consequences of ignoring the imperative of racial justice in health policy making. From the beginning it was clear: the drivers of community spread meant that COVID-19 would disproportionately sicken, disable, and kill minority Americans, would cut a major path of destruction through minority communities, and would place particular stress on the health care safety net on which these communities depend. Faced with the obvious, however, the Trump administration failed these patients, communities, and providers. Officials refused to accept federal responsibility for the scope of the pandemic or for its response (Haberman and Weiland 2020), refused to use their enormous powers to relax restrictions that would broaden the reach of the programs they administered, and refused to target resources to the highest-need communities. Even when Congress appropriated resources, the administration redirected them away from where they were most needed. Throughout, the Trump administration continued to aggressively defend a policy that officials had designed "with almost surgical precision" (to borrow a phrase from a widely publicized Voting Rights Act case)[1] to punish immigrants simply for seeking aid for which they were eligible.

For this article we have selected four separate instances in which ostensibly neutral administration decisions carried enormous equity implications for minority Americans. The first was its refusal to create a special Marketplace enrollment period for millions of workers experiencing pandemic-related job losses and lacking affordable insurance, thereby leaving them to face the ravages of the virus uninsured. The second was its refusal to use the full breadth of its regulatory powers as well as special experimental and demonstration powers to enable states to enhance and strengthen Medicaid coverage and financing. The third was the administration's unrelenting defense of its "public charge" regulation (since set aside by the Biden administration), which was explicitly designed to deny permanent legal residence status to immigrants who applied for or used health care, nutrition, and housing services for which they qualified. The final example focuses on the administration's formula for allocating CARES Act emergency health care funding, which effectively moved resources away from, rather than toward, uninsured patients and the most highly stressed clinics and hospitals. (This instance is explored in greater depth elsewhere in this issue by Grogan, Lin, and Gusmano.)

We chose these specific instances because they vividly illustrate the problem of policies that, even if not the product of a specific intent to

---

1. *North Carolina State Conference of the NAACP et al. v. McCrory et al.*, 831 F.3d 204 (4th Cir. 2016), cert. den. 137 S. Ct. 1399 (2017).

discriminate on the basis of race (and arguably the public charge rule verged on a precipice of racial animus), caused extraordinary harm to minority individuals, patients, and communities by moving resources away from them during the worst public health emergency in a century. What is key is that in each case, officials had the indisputable power to make different decisions, and as a result, the inequities their actions produced were the result of their own decisions and not ones superimposed by legislative commands. Many more examples were logical candidates for inclusion, such as the administration's decision early in the pandemic to relax Medicaid nursing home preadmission and resident review screening protocols, which in turn elevated the risk of unnecessary, grossly unsafe institutionalization of disproportionately minority, severely disabled people, even as the nursing home death toll mounted (Chidambaram, Garfield, and Neuman 2020). Furthermore, this same exercise could have been replicated in an article focusing on policies with a disproportionate adverse impact on people with disabilities, such as giving states the power to reduce the scope of Medicaid coverage during the pandemic despite a clear maintenance-of-effort statutory requirement imposed as a condition of enhanced federal funding. Similarly, this analysis could have focused on examples of sex discrimination, such as suspending remote access to medication abortion drugs during the pandemic, even as access to other forms of remote prescribing was expanded.[2] The problem, in other words, is the widespread nature of health inequities depending on the definitional equity frame one uses.

Failure to Establish a Special Enrollment Period for Workers Experiencing Pandemic-Related Job Loss

The pandemic triggered enormous job loss. By April 2020, unemployment had surged to 14.7%, and by June, 17.9 million people were uninsured. As of August, the number of workers whose temporary loss of employment had moved to long-term stood at 8.1 million (Fronstin and Woodbury 2020).

Among jobs lost by June 2020, 7.7 million (fewer than half) came with employer coverage; the nature of COVID-19 meant that disappearing work disproportionately involved jobs without health benefits (Fronstin and Woodbury 2020). For example, within the accommodation and food services industry, employment fell by 30% compared to prepandemic levels, but only 25% of workers in this employment sector had employer coverage in their own name. By contrast, manufacturing job losses (a far bigger sector) reflected 10% of this sector's prepandemic job levels, but 66% of all

---

2. *Food and Drug Administration v. ACOG*, U.S., Jan. 12, 2021.

workers in this sector had health benefits in their own name. In other words, those tending to lose jobs received lower wages and were less likely to have health benefits to begin with.

Workers experiencing job loss theoretically have several options. One is to acquire coverage through another household member with employer coverage. The Urban Institute estimated that about one-third of those experiencing job loss would do so (Banthin et al. 2020). Another option is to purchase COBRA coverage to extend their own employer coverage. However, this option obviously is limited to those with employer coverage to begin with and is extremely costly, since it comes without employer contributions. In 2019 family coverage averaged $20,599 (Pollitz et al. 2020). (The 2021 American Rescue Plan would ultimately provide short-term relief with respect to the COBRA affordability problem by subsidizing laid-off workers' premiums for several months.)

A third option is to turn to one of the Affordable Care Act's "insurance affordability programs," meaning the subsidized Marketplace, Medicaid, or the Children's Health Insurance Program (CHIP). This option is more affordable for people whose incomes have vanished. Whereas one month of self-only COBRA insurance averaged $599 in 2019, laid-off workers with $15,000 in annual income who lost jobs and health benefits and turned to the Marketplace for coverage would pay $26 in monthly premiums for a single adult and $77 per month for a single adult with $20,000 in household income (Pollitz et al. 2020). Medicaid would be virtually free. As of fall 2020, 36 states plus the District of Columbia provided Medicaid to working-age adults with incomes up to 138% of the federal poverty level; two more states (Oklahoma and Missouri) had adopted but not yet implemented the adult Medicaid expansion (KFF 2020).

Medicaid enrollment is available at any time coverage is needed. By contrast, the Marketplace works according to traditional insurance norms. To avoid adverse selection, Marketplace rules limit enrollment to an annual open period and to certain specifically designated "special enrollment periods" (SEPs) that avert the temptation to buy insurance only when health care is needed. Loss of workplace or other health benefits qualifies as a SEP, but simply losing one's job ordinarily does not. Individuals who have an immediate need for coverage (e.g., they fear facing a pandemic without insurance) but do not qualify for special enrollment periods must wait until the next annual open enrollment period. Open enrollment typically takes place in the fall both in states that operate their own Marketplaces and in the federal Marketplace (HealthCare.gov 2020). Thus, people who lost their jobs early in the pandemic but had no coverage when they were working would have had to wait until the fall open enrollment period unless they were poor enough to qualify for Medicaid and fortunate enough to live in one of the states that offered coverage under the ACA expansion. The SEP for people losing job-based benefits was not available to these newly unemployed people.

The obvious answer was to create a SEP covering all persons experiencing pandemic job loss and in need of Marketplace coverage. Indeed, the Affordable Care Act gives the Department of Health and Human Services (HHS) Secretary broad SEP designation powers,[3] and federal implementing regulations in fact authorize the creation of SEPs for "exceptional circumstances."[4] HHS thus had the power to recognize a pandemic-related SEP to aid all people losing jobs regardless of insurance coverage status at the time of job loss. Equity-mindful policy making would have led to such a decision, which would have been especially important to lower-wage workers, who are disproportionately members of racial or ethnic minority groups and significantly less likely to have job-based health coverage (Kinder and Ross 2020). Insurers did not resist such a policy; indeed, insurers have experienced record profits during the pandemic (Abelson 2020) and could have managed the additional exposure.

Given the sensibility of a SEP linked to pandemic job loss, 12 of the 13 states that operate their own Marketplaces (all but Idaho) designated a pandemic SEP (Lueck and Broaddus 2020). But Trump administration officials refused to do so, rejecting an option that they had full power to pursue and leaving millions of laid-off workers across 38 states without access to subsidized insurance in the event they needed it (Schwab, Giovannelli, and Lucia 2020). When asked at the end of March why such a policy would not be pursued, one federal official stated that the administration was "exploring other options" (Luthi 2020). These "other options" never materialized, of course; indeed, as discussed below, the administration compounded this early failure with later decisions to redirect resources meant to keep providers financially afloat, away from those providers disproportionately likely to treat uninsured patients because of their location in, and service to, poor communities.

Refusal to Fully Employ Medicaid Expansion Powers

As the scale of what the nation was facing became clear, what to do about the uninsured rose to the forefront. A large and growing number of people continued to lack health insurance, (Broaddus and Aron-Dine 2020), and

---

3. Affordable Care Act, Pub. L. No. 111-148, 124 Stat. 119 (2010), § 1311, codified at 42 U.S.C. § 18031.
4. 45 C.F.R. § 155.420.

despite progress in ending racial disparities in insurance coverage, the uninsured remain disproportionately Black, Brown, and Native American (Artiga, Orgera, and Damico 2020). In 2018 uninsured rates for Hispanic Americans stood at 19%, more than double the rate for Whites (8%); among Black Americans, the uninsured rate stood at 11% (KFF 2020).

The lack of access to Marketplace coverage represents one aspect of the problem, but another is the ongoing failure of at least a dozen states to adopt the ACA Medicaid expansion. In these nonexpansion states, eligibility for Marketplace premium subsidies begins at 100% of poverty; people with incomes below this threshold are caught in a coverage gap—ineligible for federally subsidized insurance. The remaining nonexpansion states are disproportionately concentrated in the South, meaning that the people caught in the gap are disproportionately Black. (Garfield, Orgera, and Damico 2020).

The problems that confront the uninsured poor also confront health care providers, such as community health centers, public hospitals, and mission-driven hospitals that serve poor populations and depend heavily on Medicaid as a source of revenue. (Cunningham et al. 2016; Rosenbaum et al. 2019). These providers disproportionately serve minority patients, are located in the poorest communities, and have the narrowest operating margins (Barnett, Mehrotra, and Landon 2020), and thus were heavily affected by the loss of revenue for non-COVID–related care compounded by the high costs of treating COVID patients and adapting to operating during a pandemic (Ollove 2020). For example, by the week of April 10, COVID costs rose and cumulative patient revenue losses reached $372 million at the nation's community health centers; by October, cumulative health center revenue losses exceeded an estimated $3.2 billion, 10% of annual health center operating revenue for the year (RCHN Community Health Foundation 2020).

Medicaid's unique structure as an insurer governed by public health rules rather than traditional insurance norms gives it the power to adapt to public health emergencies (Rosenbaum 2020a, Rosenbaum 2020b), with the potential to expand eligibility and coverage and increase financial support for Medicaid-dependent providers. Medicaid has played this role in past emergencies, and thus the imperative to deploy its resources grew once again so that states could ramp up eligibility, coverage, and direct funding support.

Federal policy offers four Medicaid flexibility pathways. First, states can amend their state Medicaid plans to take fuller advantage of existing federal options to expand eligibility, broaden covered benefits, simplify program management, and enhance provider payment (Manatt Health 2020; Musumeci et al. 2020). Second, Congress can amend federal Medicaid law to create new state flexibility options while enhancing federal funding levels. Third, the HHS Secretary can use his special emergency public health powers under section 1135 of the Social Security Act to give states certain flexibilities where provider enrollment and payment are concerned (CMS n.d.). This power does not enable expanded eligibility flexibility, however.

Fourth, using special Social Security Act demonstration powers, known as section 1115 powers, the secretary can develop and approve demonstrations that permit states to test Medicaid in ways not otherwise allowed under existing law as long as the Secretary finds that a demonstration is likely to promote Medicaid's core purpose of providing medical assistance to those who need it (Manatt Health 2020; Musumeci et al. 2020; Rosenbaum et al. 2016). Normally 1115 experiments are guided by strict budget neutrality rules that limit the ability to expand programs. But the concept of budget neutrality is a creature of administrative policy and not mandated by statute, and both the Trump administration and prior administrations have used their power to shape budget neutrality principles to accommodate broader innovations, especially during public health emergencies. For example, the Bush administration waived budget neutrality to enable Louisiana to expand Medicaid in the wake of Hurricane Katrina, allow New York to broaden its program following the World Trade Center attacks, and effectuate added benefits needed to treat lead poisoning in Flint (MAC Learning Collaborative 2018; Rosenbaum 2016, 2020c).

It was clear that broadening Medicaid eligibility would not be part of the initial congressional response. The Families First Coronavirus Response Act (FFCRA),[5] enacted on March 18, added a new, fully federally funded Medicaid uninsured option and enhanced federal Medicaid funding; however, the uninsured option was limited to testing only, and the FFCRA funding enhancement was limited to existing populations and conditioned on states' agreement not to reduce benefits, increase premiums or cost sharing, or terminate coverage for program enrollees (Eichner 2020). In other words, FFCRA created no new temporary option to extend Medicaid to the uninsured for treatment and recovery costs. (The HEROES Act, passed by the House of Representatives in May 2020, contained this broader coverage flexibility [Youdelman 2020], but this change never passed Congress.)

---

5. Pub. L. No. 116-127, 134 Stat. 178 (2020).

Several states, most notably Washington State, immediately sought Medicaid eligibility expansion flexibility through 1115 as well as the ability to adopt more generous coverage and payment rules coupled with generous funding forgiveness for essential providers (Rosenbaum and Handley 2020). These changes lay beyond the reach of 1135 but had ample 1115 precedent. But despite calls from states (NAMD 2020) to allow an expanded Medicaid response coupled with more generous budget neutrality rules, the administration refused to do so. Indeed, in the midst of the pandemic, the administration instead sought US Supreme Court review of an appeals court decision barring HHS from allowing states to reduce Medicaid eligibility through work experiments (Rosenbaum et al. 2020), even though such reductions could not possibly have occurred during the pandemic because of the FFCRA maintenance of effort rule. The administration took matters a step further, issuing a rule that enabled states accepting FFCRA funding enhancements (all states) to begin eliminating enrolled people and reducing coverage despite clear statutory language to the contrary (CMS 2020).

Refusal to Suspend the Public Charge Rule during the Pandemic

Being classified as a "public charge" constitutes a basis for denying immigrants admission into the United States or the ability to become permanent legal residents. The Immigration and Nationality Act does not define the term *public charge*,[6] but, historically, the term has signified someone who is not self-sufficient and depends on the government for support.[7]

Guidance issued by the Clinton administration in 1999 following enactment of the Personal Responsibility and Work Opportunity Reconciliation Act[8] and the Illegal Immigration Reform and Immigrant Responsibility Act limited dependence on government support to evidence that an individual "is primarily dependent on the government for subsistence" as evidenced by either "(i) receipt of public cash assistance for income maintenance or (ii) institutionalization for long-term care at government expense."[9] The guidance thus excluded from its definition of "primarily dependent" other public benefits designed to supplement basic income, such as Medicaid for health care needs other than long-term institutionalization, Supplemental

---

6. Pub. L. No. 89-236, 79 Stat. 911 (1965).
7. *State of New York et al. v. United States Department of Homeland Security* (2d Cir., 2020).
8. PRWORA, Pub. L. No. 104-193, 110 Stat. 2105 (1996); Pub. L. No. 104-208, 110 Stat. 3009-546 (1996).
9. 64 Fed. Reg. (1999).

Nutrition Assistance Program (SNAP) food assistance benefits, and public housing. Additionally, the 1999 guidance applied a "totality of circumstances" test governing public charge determinations that explicitly instructed immigration officials that neither current nor past receipt of cash welfare would automatically make an individual a public charge.

In 2019, as part of its broad, sustained attack on immigration and immigrants generally, the Trump administration issued a rule that sweeps away this narrow approach to public charge determinations.[10] Under the final rule, the concept of public charge was no longer confined to primary dependence on the government for subsistence. Instead, receipt of "one or more public benefits ... for more than 12 months in the aggregate within any 36-month period" could qualify someone as a public charge. Furthermore, the benefits to be counted in making such a determination included both monetizable (i.e., cash welfare) and non-monetizable assistance, including many forms of Medicaid along with SNAP assistance and public housing supports. The 12-month durational threshold was "deceptive" (in the words of one court, *New York v. Department of Homeland Security*), since it was to be applied cumulatively. For example, an injured worker who needed Medicaid and SNAP during her 7-month recovery period would exceed the 12-month test by 2 months (2 "benefit months" × 7 months). The rule intensified the impact of this dramatically enhanced definition of what constitutes public assistance by intensifying an adjudication process to predict who in the future might be a public charge (Ku 2019) using certain factors: age (younger than 18 or older than 61), health status, family status, financial status including income and assets, and education and skills. Under this process, being a child or older than 61 would be a strike against the applicant. Having a medical condition "likely to require extensive medical treatment or institutionalization or that will interfere with the agency's ability to provide care for himself or herself, to attend school or to work" would be a strike against the applicant. Being a member of a larger family would be a strike, since larger families are more likely to be poor. A similar strike would be low income or limited education. In its final rule, the administration dismissed as speculative and beside the point extensive evidence in the administrative record (including previous government-sponsored studies) regarding the impact of sanctions against immigrants who use public benefits.[11] With a flourish, the administration asserted that the impact of its "chilling effects" policy, as it is known, was not its problem:

10. 84 Fed. Reg. 41292 (August 14, 2019).
11. 84 Fed. Reg. 41292 (August 14, 2019) at 41310–41313.

DHS acknowledges that individuals subject to this rule may decline to enroll in, or may choose to disenroll from, public benefits for which they may be eligible. . . . However, DHS has authority to take past, current, and likely future receipt of public benefits into account, even where it may ultimately result in discouraging aliens from receiving public benefits. Although individuals may reconsider their receipt of public benefits as defined by this rule in light of future immigration consequences, this rule does not prohibit an alien from obtaining a public benefit for which he or she is eligible. DHS expects that aliens seeking lawful permanent resident status or nonimmigrant status in the United States will make purposeful and well-informed decisions commensurate with the immigration status they are seeking.[12]

Within months of its adoption, research documented the impact of the rule—an impact that extended into the pandemic period (Bernstein et al. 2020).

Upon publication, numerous states and nonprofit organizations launched a nationwide effort to halt the rule from taking effect. The effort failed, in one case because of a ruling on the merits in the administration's favor, and in other cases because, despite wins at the appellate level, the US Supreme Court allowed the rule to go into effect while appeals were pending (Parmet 2020). The court's decision preceded the public emergency declaration by three weeks.

Shortly after the emergency declaration, and with the Supreme Court's permission, the New York plaintiffs returned to court, arguing that the injunction should be reconsidered, given the materially changed circumstances wrought by the pandemic and the far greater threat now posed by the rule's chilling effect. Indeed, the danger was not lost on the administration. Having included an emergency exception in its own rule, the administration acknowledged these changed circumstances and in March posted an obscure alert allowing the use of certain public benefits related to COVID-19 testing and treatment (USCIS 2020).

That this notice failed to mitigate the impact of the rule was made clear by the July 2020 federal trial court decision in response to the New York plaintiffs' renewed effort to halt the rule. Although this decision also was stayed on appeal, its conclusions nonetheless underscored the gravity of clinging to the rule during the worst communicable disease pandemic in a century and the meaninglessness of the administration's nominal effort at an informal exception policy. Writing that the rule "has demonstrably failed

12. 84 Fed. Reg. 41312–41313.

the first real world test of its application," the court found that the policy "deters immigrants from seeking testing and treatment for COVID-19" based on testimony from physicians and others who "have all witnessed immigrants refusing to enroll in Medicaid or other publicly funded health coverage, or forgoing testing and treatment for COVID-19, out of fear that accepting such insurance or care will increase their risk of being labeled a 'public charge.'" The court further found that the administration's informal guidance was "unlikely to remedy Plaintiffs' harms considering its limited scope," since immigrants would have no means of showing that they had enrolled solely to receive COVID-19 treatment, would be penalized for using Medicaid to treat other serious health conditions during enrollment, and, indeed, would be penalized simply for enrolling.[13]

In sum, the administration could have formally suspended a rule whose individual and public health impact was obvious from the start, even to the administration. It chose not to do so.

Failure to Target Emergency Health Care Provider Relief

Through laws enacted in March and April, Congress appropriated a total of $175 billion in emergency health care relief. Funding came principally through the Coronavirus Aid, Relief, and Economic Security (CARES) Act.[14] Additional emergency health care funding came through the Coronavirus Preparedness Response Supplemental Appropriations Act,[15] FFCRA, and the Paycheck Protection Program and Health Care Enhancement Act.[16]

Congress allocated the largest share of total emergency health care funding to HHS. The largest share of this funding was intended to go to hospital relief, although community-based health programs and providers also were eligible to receive funding. While the HHS secretary was given broad discretion over how funding would be allocated, it was also the case that the fund was to serve two principal purposes: to offset the cost of paying for COVID-19–related testing and treatment for uninsured people, and to assist providers (principally hospitals) that had experienced high revenue loss as non–COVID-19 care payments disappeared.

Within weeks, serious problems with the administration's approach to implementation emerged. Of the first $72.4 billion in fund distributions,

13. *New York v. United States Department of Homeland Security*, 20 WL 4347264 (July 29, 2020).

14. Pub. L. No. 116-136 (March 27, 2020).

15. Pub. L. No. 116-123 (March 6, 2020).

16. Pub. L. No. 116-139 (April 24, 2020).

the administration allocated $50 billion to Medicare-participating providers based on total net revenue from all payer sources. This formula meant that emergency government funding favored hospitals with a higher level of private health insurance revenue, larger operating margins, and less uncompensated care (Schwartz and Damico 2020). As a result, the initial tranche of funding flowed toward financially stronger hospitals operating in more affluent communities and away from the hardest-hit hospitals most dependent on public funding, operating with the narrowest financial margins, showing the highest uninsured rates, and serving the poorest communities with elevated minority residential rates (Mann and Mauser 2020).

The formula thus had a disparate impact on communities most in need of protection (Kakani et al. 2020). Indeed, the government's allocation methodology tracked a separate algorithm previously used to determine patients in need of medical monitoring for complex conditions that turned out to discriminate in practice against Black patients (Bass and Tozzi 2020). The administration's response to this mounting evidence was to dismiss concerns, arguing that other allocation methods "would have taken much longer to implement" (Bass and Tozzi 2020). So serious were the risks caused by the allocation formula that even in a period of intense congressional partisanship, leading senators from both parties wrote the HHS secretary "to share [their] serious concerns" about the "delay in disbursing funds from the Emergency Fund for Medicaid-dependent providers" that in turn "could also severely hamper their ability to continue to serve as essential providers" (US Congress 2020).

In response to this outcry over its general formula, HHS modified the fund to release approximately $60 billion in additional relief to certain targeted providers: hospitals located in "high impact areas"; hospitals serving rural populations; skilled nursing facilities; safety net hospitals; and tribal hospitals, clinics, and urban health centers (HHS 2020). Although this correction provided some relief, by HHS's own figures, allocations to high-need providers in high-need communities represented the minority of the total $175 billion Emergency Fund.

Recall, moreover, that in refusing to establish a broad SEP for workers facing pandemic-related job loss, the administration noted that it was "exploring other options." These "other options" essentially turned out to amount to an allocation of $1.3 billion of the $175 billion for payments to hospitals and other health care providers for costs associated with caring for the uninsured. In other words, despite promises to explore "other options," by early fall the administration had allocated 0.7% of the fund to offsetting the cost of treating uninsured patients, whose total cost had been estimated at between $13.9 billion and $41.8 billion (Levitt, Schwartz, and Lopez 2020).

Furthermore, the problems extended well beyond the size of the fund in relation to need. The fund is administered as largesse rather than as a government program; that is, hospitals can choose to participate and can select who receives help; they are under no obligation to make its existence known to patients (Rosenbaum 2020a). The administration also imposed strict limitations on which costs qualify for payment, meaning that hospitals treating patients with COVID-19–related complications experienced high numbers of claims rejections (Schwartz and Tolbert 2020). Patients have been billed for care that should have qualified for payment, and as a result of payment restrictions, hospitals report up to 40% of billed claims have gone unpaid, even when treatment was urgently needed for common complications of COVID-19 or co-occurring conditions such as sepsis (Ruoff 2020).

Ultimately, the uninsured claims fund emerged as yet another example of deliberate choices, in the face of broad discretion over the design of a resource allocation strategy, that, while ostensibly neutral, had a racially identifiable impact. The allocation formula built on a model already noted for its discriminatory effects that disfavored poor providers in poor communities and invested virtually nothing in uninsured patients. Even the funds that were targeted to uninsured claims fell far short of the limited impact they might have had because participation remained voluntary and the program lacked procedures for ensuring that patients and families were informed of the existence of such funds and had an opportunity to apply. Ironically, a workable model for these basic due-process safeguards readily exists, found in the community benefit regulations that govern operations of nonprofit hospitals claiming tax-exempt status (IRS n.d.). The administration ignored the model in favor of a dysfunctional, grossly unfair approach that then became an excuse for not doing more for the uninsured.

Discussion

In the midst of a once-in-a-century public health emergency, discretion to the executive branch is absolutely vital. Congress can rapidly appropriate funding and enact broad-brush legislative reforms. Inevitably it falls to the executive branch to rapidly implement reforms. As these examples illustrate, however, absent health equity mindfulness, there is no real check on the formulation of unjust policy. The Administrative Procedure Act

(APA) guarantees the public the right to notice of agency policy reforms and the opportunity to comment, and policies must be reasonable and must take public comment periods into account. Nonetheless, in accordance with the precepts of the APA, the courts are hesitant to substitute their own judgment for that of agencies with expertise, and they assign the responsibility for formulating administrative policy to the executive branch (*Food and Drug Administration v. ACOG*). Thus, in the absence of a clear policy of equity mindfulness, agencies can pursue policies that exacerbate rather than mitigate racial inequities.

These relatively straightforward examples also point to what an equity-mindful approach to executive policy making might have looked like: a special Marketplace enrollment period covering all people experiencing pandemic-related job loss, not only those who also lost health benefits; full use of Medicaid policy making powers to invite and approve public health emergency demonstrations expanding eligibility, coverage, and payments for the duration of the pandemic and a reasonable recovery period; an immediate suspension of rules already shown to be explosively harmful to immigrants (of course, in an equity-mindful world, these rules never would have been promulgated to begin with); and an emergency health care funding allocation process that would have favored the highest-need providers and communities and would have afforded patients and families a clear means of understanding the availability of help and applying for assistance.

The Trump administration did not simply ignore readily available evidence of the people and communities most endangered and most in need of health care supports; its policies truly appear to have targeted these people and communities with "almost surgical precision"—a phrase remarkable in its accuracy. The choices were so blind to their consequences as to border on intentional harm, not merely harmful effect. But to reach the level of intent, actual evidence of a deliberate decision to discriminate would be needed; circumstantial evidence does not suffice.

There is reason for hope. The Biden administration positioned itself to bring a dramatically different approach to executive policy making, one that elevates the importance of health equity as a guiding principle of implementation design and execution. The early evidence of this new direction could be seen in the administration's announced COVID-19 vaccination plan, which, as a core element, emphasized a robust, nationwide network of access points in communities of color (Ollstein 2021). Other examples followed, shown in the administration's decision to rapidly establish a special Marketplace enrollment period for people experiencing pandemic-related job loss as well as in the American Rescue Plan envisioned by the president (Tankersley and Crowley 2021) and ultimately enacted by Congress.[17]

But the fact that the Biden administration acted in a fundamentally different manner is not the end of things. Two matters require attention. First, it is imperative to fund a full evaluation of how the Trump administration's policy choices affected access to health care among minority patients and by minority communities. This process has begun as the studies cited in this article suggest. But we need far more extensive research if we are to avoid repeating the errors of the COVID-19 response. Of course, the country needs to fully understand how the pandemic affected minority individuals and families and communities of color; but we already knew that these people and communities would be most heavily affected.

Even more importantly in terms of new knowledge, policy makers need to understand how specific policies either mitigated or worsened the on-the-ground conditions. What were the characteristics of the people forced to endure a pandemic without health insurance, and how many more would have been insured had the administration taken steps to broaden Marketplace and Medicaid coverage? How many avoidable deaths did the pandemic produce as a result of inadequate access to rapid, intensive care? How did immigrant communities fare, and how did failure to lift the public charge rule entirely affect access to services? How did health care providers, serving different communities, fare during the pandemic in terms of service capabilities, and what have been their experiences in regaining operational strength?

Second, it is important to consider whether, as part of health policy making, it is time to formalize the aspirational goal of ending structural racism in policy making itself. Today, when rules are promulgated, agencies must consider their impact on the economy, state and local governments, small businesses, and other stakeholders. Is it not time to recognize an additional analytic step—a formal health equity assessment as part of the policy-making process that would cover both the formal rulemaking process and the development of the type of large-scale informal guidance that may be exempt from full APA notice and comment requirements but that nonetheless drives so much policy? The $175 billion provider relief fund is just such guidance—an obscure website whose contents were developed entirely behind closed doors, without any public consideration of its potential effects; indeed, people, communities, and health care providers felt its effects only after tens of billions of dollars in federal funding had flowed out.

---

17. Pub. L. 117-2 (2021)

Recognizing the speed with which public health emergency responses must happen and with which public policies so often must be formulated more generally, is it not nonetheless time to undertake the type of rapid analytic step so frequently used in the policy making process to fully consider health equity effects before policies are adopted? This is not an absurd suggestion. Adding such a step is consistent with the use of predictive modeling techniques typically brought to bear on large-scale policy decisions by the Office of Management and Budget or the Congressional Budget Office (Huntley and Miller 2009). Determining the effects of policies on large population groups is no less urgent than considering their impact on small businesses.

Adding such a formal prospective evaluation step to health policy making is consistent with the literature on structural racism, which aims to fundamentally alter the ways in which policy makers create solutions to social health problems. Moreover, it is entirely consistent with US civil rights law. This is especially so in the case of health policy making. Section 1557 (42 U.S.C. § 18116) of the Affordable Care Act extended the federal legal prohibition against discrimination based on race, color, and national origin (as well as laws prohibiting discrimination based on age, sex, and handicap) to the entire health system. Furthermore, section 1557 binds not only federal funding recipients but also the executive branch as well. Given the lessons learned during COVID-19, it seems only logical to take 1557 to its fullest logical extent and add a formal process of health equity measurement to the agency health policy making process itself.

■ ■ ■

Sara Rosenbaum is the Harold and Jane Hirsh Professor of Health Law and Policy and founding chair of the Department of Health Policy at George Washington University's Milken Institute School of Public Health. She is a member of the National Academies of Sciences, Engineering, and Medicine; has served on the CDC's Director's Advisory Committee and Advisory Committee on Immunization Practice; and was a founding commissioner of Congress's Medicaid and CHIP Payment and Access Commission (MACPAC), which she chaired from January 2016 through April 2017. She has devoted her career to health justice for medically underserved populations and is the 2020 recipient of the National Academy of Medicine's Adam Yarmolinsky Medal, awarded for distinguished service to a member from a discipline outside the health and medical sciences.
sarar@gwu.edu

Morgan Handley is a senior research associate with the Department of Health Policy at George Washington University's Milken Institute School of Public Health. Her work focuses on Medicaid, health reform, and medically underserved populations.

Rebecca Morris is a PhD candidate in public policy and public administration and a research associate with the Department of Health Policy at George Washington University's Milken Institute School of Public Health. Her work focuses on Medicaid, behavioral health, and health reform.

Maria Casoni is a senior research associate with the Department of Health Policy and Management at George Washington University's Milken Institute School of Public Health, where she has focused on law and policy issues relating to the Affordable Care Act, Medicaid, and other federal and state programs.

References

Abelson, Reed. 2020. "Major US Health Insurers Report Big Profits, Benefiting from the Pandemic." *New York Times*, August 5. www.nytimes.com/2020/08/05/health /covid-insurance-profits.html?smid=em-share.

Artiga, Samantha, Kendal Orgera, and Anthony Damico. 2020. "Changes in Health Coverage by Race and Ethnicity since the ACA, 2010–2018." Kaiser Family Foundation, March 5. www.kff.org/racial-equity-and-health-policy/issue-brief /changes-in-health-coverage-by-race-and-ethnicity-since-the-aca-2010-2018/.

Banthin, Jessica, Michael Simpson, Matthew Buettgens, Linda J. Blumberg, and Robin Wang. 2020. "Changes in Health Insurance Coverage Due to the COVID-19 Recession." Urban Institute, July 13. www.urban.org/research/publication/changes -health-insurance-coverage-due-covid-19-recession.

Barnett, Michael L., Ateev Mehrotra, and Bruce E. Landon. 2020. "Covid-19 and the Upcoming Financial Crisis in Health Care." *New England Journal of Medicine Catalyst*, April 29. catalyst.nejm.org/doi/full/10.1056/CAT.20.0153.

Bass, Dina, and John Tozzi. 2020. "US Covid Funding Flaw Shortchanges Hospitals in Black Communities." *Bloomberg*, September 10. www.bloomberg.com/news/articles /2020-09-10/u-s-covid-funding-flaw-shortchanges-hospitals-in-black-communities.

Berkowitz, Seth A., Crystal Wiley Cené, and Avik Chatterjee. 2020. "Covid-19 and Health Equity—Time to Think Big." *New England Journal of Medicine* 383, no. 12: e76.

Bernstein, Hamutal, Dulce Gonzalez, Michael Karpman, and Stephen Zuckerman. 2020. "Amid Confusion over the Public Charge Rule, Immigrant Families Continued Avoiding Public Benefits in 2019." Urban Institute, May 18. www.urban.org /research/publication/amid-confusion-over-public-charge-rule-immigrant-families -continued-avoiding-public-benefits-2019.

Biden, Joseph R. 2021. "Executive Order on Ensuring an Equitable Pandemic Response and Recovery." January 21. www.whitehouse.gov/briefing-room/presidential-actions /2021/01/21/executive-order-ensuring-an-equitable-pandemic-response-and-recovery/.

Blumenthal, David, Elizabeth J. Fowler, Melinda Abrams, and Sara R. Collins. 2020. "Covid-19—Implications for the Health Care System." *New England Journal of Medicine* 383, no. 15: 1483–88.

Broaddus, Matt, and Aviva Aron-Dine. 2020. "Uninsured Rate Rose Again in 2019, Further Eroding Earlier Progress." Center on Budget and Policy Priorities, September 15. www.cbpp.org/research/health/uninsured-rate-rose-again-in-2019-further-eroding -earlier-progress#: ∼ :text=Some%209.2%20percent%20of%20Americans,accor ding%20to%20the%20ACS%20data.

Byrd, W. Michael, and Linda A. Clayton. 2001. *An American Health Dilemma: A Medical History of African Americans and the Problem of Race, Beginnings to 1900*. New York: Routledge.

Chidambaram, Priya, Rachel Garfield, and Tricia Neuman. 2020. "COVID-19 Has Claimed the Lives of 100,000 Long-Term Care Residents and Staff." Kaiser Family Foundation, November 25. www.kff.org/policy-watch/covid-19-has-claimed-the -lives-of-100000-long-term-care-residents-and-staff/.

CMS (Centers for Medicare and Medicaid Services). n.d. "1135 Waiver—At a Glance." www.cms.gov/Medicare/Provider-Enrollment-and-Certification/SurveyCertEmerg Prep/Downloads/1135-Waivers-At-A-Glance.pdf (accessed April 20, 2021).

CMS (Centers for Medicare and Medicaid Services). 2020. "Fourth COVID-19 Interim Final Rule with Comment Period (IFC-4)." October 28. www.cms.gov/newsroom/fact -sheets/fourth-covid-19-interim-final-rule-comment-period-ifc-4.

Cunningham, Peter, Robin Rudowitz, Katherine Young, Rachel Garfield, and Julia Foutz. 2016. "Understanding Medicaid Hospital Payments and the Impact of Recent Policy Changes." Kaiser Family Foundation, June 9. www.kff.org/report-section /understanding-medicaid-hospital-payments-and-the-impact-of-recent-policy -changes-issue-brief/.

Egede, Leonard E., and Rebekah J. Walker. 2020. "Structural Racism, Social Risk Factors, and COVID-19—A Dangerous Convergence for Black Americans." *New England Journal of Medicine* 383, no. 12: e77.

Eichner, Hannah. 2020. "Top Ten List: Maintenance of Effort Requirement Compli- ance." National Health Law Program, June. healthlaw.org/wp-content/uploads/2020 /06/Top-10-MOE-Final.pdf.

Figueroa, Jose F., Rishi K. Wadhera, Dennis Lee, Robert W. Yeh, and Benjamin D. Sommers. 2020. "Community-Level Factors Associated with Racial and Ethnic Disparities in COVID-19 Rates in Massachusetts." *Health Affairs* 39, no. 9: 1624–32.

Fronstin, Paul, and Stephen A. Woodbury. 2020. "How Many Americans Have Lost Jobs with Employer Health Coverage during the Pandemic?" Commonwealth Fund, October 7. www.commonwealthfund.org/publications/issue-briefs/2020/oct /how-many-lost-jobs-employer-coverage-pandemic.

Garfield, Rachel, Kendal Orgera, and Anthony Damico. 2020. "The Coverage Gap: Uninsured Poor Adults in States That Do Not Expand Medicaid." Kaiser Family Foundation, January 14. www.kff.org/medicaid/issue-brief/the-coverage-gap -uninsured-poor-adults-in-states-that-do-not-expand-medicaid/.

Haberman, Maggie, and Noah Weiland. 2020. "Inside the Coronavirus Response: A Case Study in the White House under Trump." *New York Times*, March 16. www.nytimes .com/2020/03/16/us/politics/kushner-trump-coronavirus.html?smid=em-share.

HealthCare.gov. 2020. "Getting Health Coverage outside Open Enrollment Enroll in or Change 2020 Plans—Only with a Special Enrollment Period." HealthCare.gov. www.healthcare.gov/coverage-outside-open-enrollment/special-enrollment-period/ (accessed October 16, 2020).

HHS (US Department of Health and Human Services). 2020. "CARES Act Provider Relief Fund: General Information." October 22. www.hhs.gov/coronavirus/cares -act-provider-relief-fund/general-information/index.html#targeted.

Huntley, Jonathan, and Eric Miller. 2009. "An Evaluation of CBO Forecasts." Congressional Budget Office Working Paper Series, August. www.cbo.gov/sites/default /files/111th-congress-2009-2010/workingpaper/2009-02_0.pdf.

IOM (Institute of Medicine). 2003. *Unequal Treatment: Confronting Racial and Ethnic Disparities in Health Care.* Washington, DC: National Academies Press. doi.org/10.17226/12875.

IRS (Internal Revenue Service). n.d. "Financial Assistance Policies." www.irs.gov /charities-non-profits/financial-assistance-policies-faps (accessed April 20, 2021).

Kakani, Pragya, Amitabh Chandra, Sendhil Mullainathan, and Ziad Obermeyer. 2020. "Allocation of COVID-19 Relief Funding to Disproportionately Black Counties." *Journal of the American Medical Association* 324, no. 10: 1000–1003.

KFF (Kaiser Family Foundation). 2020. "Status of State Medicaid Expansion Decisions: Interactive Map." October 21. www.kff.org/medicaid/issue-brief/status-of -state-medicaid-expansion-decisions-interactive-map/.

Kinder, Molly, and Martha Ross. 2020. "Reopening America: Low-Wage Workers Have Suffered Badly from COVID-19 So Policymakers Should Focus on Equity." Brookings Institution, June 23. www.brookings.edu/research/reopening-america -low-wage-workers-have-suffered-badly-from-covid-19-so-policymakers-should -focus-on-equity/.

Ku, Leighton. 2019. "Declaration of Leighton Ku, PhD, MPH, in *La Clinica de la Raza et al. v. Donald J. Trump et al.*" National Health Law Program, September 1. healthlaw.org/resource/declaration-of-leighton-ku-in-la-clinica-de-la-raza-v-trump/.

Levitt, Larry, Karyn Schwartz, and Eric Lopez. 2020. "Estimated Cost of Treating the Uninsured Hospitalized with COVID-19." Kaiser Family Foundation, April 7. www .kff.org/coronavirus-covid-19/issue-brief/estimated-cost-of-treating-the-uninsured -hospitalized-with-covid-19/.

Lueck, Sarah, and Matthew Broaddus. 2020. "Emergency Special Enrollment Period Would Boost Health Coverage Access at a Critical Time." Center on Budget and Policy Priorities, July 30. www.cbpp.org/research/health/emergency-special-enroll ment-period-would-boost-health-coverage-access-at-a-critical.

Luthi, Susannah. 2020. "Trump Rejects Obamacare Special Enrollment Period amid Pandemic." *Politico*, March 31. www.politico.com/news/2020/03/31/trump-obama care-coronavirus-157788.

MAC (Medicaid and CHIP) Learning Collaborative. 2018. "Role of Medicaid and CHIP in Responding to Public Health Crises and Disasters." August 13. www .medicaid.gov/state-resource-center/downloads/mac-learning-collaboratives/role -of-medicaid-crises-and-disasters.pdf.

Manatt Health. 2020. "Targeted Options for Increasing Medicaid Payment to Providers during COVID-19 Crisis." State Health and Value Strategies, August 26. www .shvs.org/medicaid-enhanced-provider-payment-strategies/.

Mann, Cindy, and Gayle E. Mauser. 2020. "COVID-19 Relief Needed to Keep Medicaid Community-Based Providers Afloat." Commonwealth Fund (blog), October 5. www.commonwealthfund.org/blog/2020/covid-19-relief-needed-keep-medicaid -community-based-providers-afloat.

Matthew, Dayna Bowen. 2015. *Just Medicine: A Cure for Racial Inequality in American Health Care*. New York: New York University Press.

Michener, Jamila. 2019. "Policy Feedback in a Racialized Polity." *Policy Studies Journal* 47, no. 2: 423–50.

Musumeci, MaryBeth, Robin Rudowtiz, Elizabeth Hinton, Rachel Dolan, and Olivia Pham. 2020. "Options to Support Medicaid Providers in Response to COVID-19." Kaiser Family Foundation, June 17. www.kff.org/coronavirus-covid-19/issue-brief /options-to-support-medicaid-providers-in-response-to-covid-19/#:~:text=States% 20have%20taken%20a%20number,and%20Section%201115%20demonstration% 20waivers.

NAMD (National Association of Medicaid Directors). 2020. Letter from NAMD to Calder Lynch and Russ Vought. April 6. medicaiddirectors.org/wp-content/uploads /2020/04/Letter-to-CMS-and-OMB-on-retainer-payments_4_6_20_FINAL.pdf.

Ollove, Michael. 2020. "Virus Imperils Health Care Safety Net." Pew Charitable Trusts, September 1. www.pewtrusts.org/en/research-and-analysis/blogs/stateline/2020 /09/01/virus-imperils-health-care-safety-net.

Ollstein, Alice Miranda, 2021. "Biden's Covid Vaccine Plan Targets Communities of Color." *Real Clear Politics*, January 15. www.realclearpolitics.com/2021/01/15 /bidens_covid_vaccine_plan_targets_communities_of_color_533586.html.

Oppel, Richard, Robert Gebeloff, K. K. Rebecca Lai, Will Wright, and Mitch Smith. 2020. "The Fullest Look Yet at the Racial Inequity of Coronavirus." *New York Times*, July 5. www.nytimes.com/interactive/2020/07/05/us/coronavirus-latinos -african-americans-cdc-data.html.

Oppenheim, Ben, and Gavin Yamey. 2017. "Pandemics and the Poor." Brookings Institution, June 19. www.brookings.edu/blog/future-development/2017/06/19 /pandemics-and-the-poor/.

Parmet, Wendy E. 2020. "Supreme Court Allows Public Charge Rule to Take Effect While Appeals Continue." *Health Affairs Blog*, February 3. www.healthaffairs.org /do/10.1377/hblog20200131.845894/full/.

Pollitz, Karen, Matthew Rae, Cynthia Cox, Rabah Kamal, Rachel Fehr, and Greg Young. 2020. "Key Issues Related to COBRA Subsidies." Kaiser Family Foundation, May 28. www.kff.org/private-insurance/issue-brief/key-issues-related-to -cobra-subsidies/.

RCHN Community Health Foundation. 2020. "COVID 19's Impact on CHCs." October 2. www.rchnfoundation.org/?p=9218.

Rosenbaum, Sara. 2016. "Caring for Flint: Medicaid's Enduring Role in Public Health Crises." Commonwealth Fund, February 22. www.commonwealthfund.org/blog /2016/caring-flint-medicaids-enduring-role-public-health-crises.

Rosenbaum, Sara. 2020a. "In the Pandemic, Patients Need Health Insurance, Not a Hospital 'Claims Reimbursement' Fund." *Milbank Quarterly*, May 1. www.milbank .org/quarterly/opinions/in-the-pandemic-patients-need-health-insurance-not-a -hospital-claims-reimbursement-fund/.

Rosenbaum, Sara. 2020b. "Medicaid and the Coronavirus: Putting the Nation's Largest Health Care First Responder to Work." Commonwealth Fund, March 9. www .commonwealthfund.org/blog/2020/medicaid-and-coronavirus-putting-nations -largest-health-care-first-responder-work.

Rosenbaum, Sara. 2020c. "Using Medicaid Waivers to Help States Manage the COVID-19 Public Health Crisis." Commonwealth Fund, March 26. www.common wealthfund.org/blog/2020/medicaid-waivers-states-covid-19.

Rosenbaum, Sara, and Morgan Handley. 2020. "Broadening Medicare's Accelerated and Advance Payment Program to Save Health Care Providers That Serve Our Most Vulnerable Populations." Commonwealth Fund, May 13. www.commonwealth fund.org/blog/2020/broadening-medicares-accelerated-and-advance-payment -program-save-health-care-providers.

Rosenbaum, Sara, Sara Schmucker, Sara Rothenberg, and Rachel Gunsalus. 2016. "How Will Section 1115 Medicaid Expansion Demonstrations Inform Federal Policy?" Commonwealth Fund, May 17. www.commonwealthfund.org/publications /issue-briefs/2016/may/how-will-section-1115-medicaid-expansion-demonstrations -inform.

Rosenbaum, Sara, Jessica Sharac, Peter Shin, and Jennifer Tolbert. 2019. "Community Health Center Financing: The Role of Medicaid and Section 330 Grant Funding Explained." Kaiser Family Foundation, March 26. www.kff.org/report-section /community-health-center-financing-the-role-of-medicaid-and-section-330-grant -funding-explained-executive-summary/.

Rosenbaum, Sara, Benjamin D. Sommers, and Nia Johnson. 2020. "As Trump Administration Seeks US Supreme Court Review, a Second Year of Results from Medicaid Work Experiments Emerges." *Health Affairs Blog*, October 19. www .healthaffairs.org/do/10.1377/hblog20201016.709593/full/.

Ruoff, Alex. 2020. "US Covid Program Leaves Uninsured with 'Bills They Can't Pay.'" *Bloomberg Government*, October 13. about.bgov.com/news/u-s-covid-program -leaves-uninsured-with-bills-they-cant-pay/#:~:text=The%20federal%20program% 20to%20pay,and%20hospitals%20with%20mounting%20bills.

Schwab, Rachel, Justin Giovannelli, and Kevin Lucia. 2020. "During the COVID-19 Crisis, State Health Insurance Marketplaces Are Working to Enroll the Uninsured." Commonwealth Fund, May 19. www.commonwealthfund.org/blog/2020/during -covid-19-crisis-state-health-insurance-marketplaces-are-working-enroll-uninsured.

Schwartz, Karyn, and Anthony Damico. 2020. "Distribution of CARES Act Funding among Hospitals." Kaiser Family Foundation, May 13. www.kff.org/coronavirus -covid-19/issue-brief/distribution-of-cares-act-funding-among-hospitals/.

Schwartz, Karyn, and Jennifer Tolbert. 2020. "Limitations of the Program for Uninsured COVID-19 Patients Raise Concerns." Kaiser Family Foundation, October 8. www.kff.org/policy-watch/limitations-of-the-program-for-uninsured-covid-19 -patients-raise-concerns/.

Selden, Thomas M., and Terceira A. Berdahl. 2020. "COVID-19 and Racial/Ethnic Disparities in Health Risk, Employment, and Household Composition: Study Examines Potential Explanations for Racial-Ethnic Disparities in COVID-19 Hospitalizations and Mortality." *Health Affairs* 39, no. 9: 1624–32.

Smith, David Barton. 1999. *Health Care Divided: Race and Healing a Nation.* Ann Arbor: University of Michigan Press.

Tankersley, Jim, and Michael Crowley. 2021."Biden Outlines $1.9 Trillion Spending Package to Combat Virus and Downturn." *New York Times*, January 14. www .nytimes.com/2021/01/14/business/economy/biden-economy.html.

US Congress. 2020. Letter from the US Congress to HHS Secretary Alex Azar. June 3. www.finance.senate.gov/imo/media/doc/060320%20Medicaid%20Provider%20 Fund%20Letter.pdf.

US House of Representatives, House Committee on Ways and Means. 2021. "Something Must Change: Inequities in US Policy and Society." Majority Staff Report, January. waysandmeans.house.gov/sites/democrats.waysandmeans.house.gov /files/documents/WMD%20Health%20and%20Economic%20Equity%20Vision_ REPORT.pdf.

USCIS (US Citizenship and Immigration Services). 2020. "Public Charge." Department of Homeland Security, US Citizenship and Immigration Services, September 22. www.uscis.gov/green-card/green-card-processes-and-procedures/public-charge.

Youdelman, Mara. 2020. "Medicaid Needs to Remain the Hero: A Summary of the HEROES Act." National Health Law Program, May. healthlaw.org/wp-content /uploads/2020/05/The-HEROES-Act-fact-sheet-FINAL.pdf.

Unsanitized and Unfair: How COVID-19 Bailout Funds Refuel Inequity in the US Health Care System

Colleen M. Grogan
University of Chicago

Yu-An Lin
National Taipei University

Michael K. Gusmano
Rutgers University

Abstract

Context: The CARES Act of 2020 allocated provider relief funds to hospitals and other providers. We investigate whether these funds were distributed in a way that responded fairly to COVID-19–related medical and financial need. The US health care system is bifurcated into the "haves" and "have nots." The health care safety net hospitals, which were already financially weak, cared for the bulk of COVID-19 cases. In contrast, the "have" hospitals suffered financially because their most profitable procedures are elective and were postponed during the COVID-19 outbreak.

Methods: To obtain relief fund data for each hospital in the United States, we started with data from the HHS website. We use the RAND Hospital Data tool to analyze how fund distributions are associated with hospital characteristics.

Findings: Our analysis reveals that the "have" hospitals with the most days of cash on hand received more funding per bed than hospitals with fewer than 50 days of cash on hand (the "have nots").

Conclusions: Despite extreme racial inequities, which COVID-19 exposed early in the pandemic, the federal government rewards those hospitals that cater to the most privileged in the United States, leaving hospitals that predominantly serve low-income people of color with less.

Keywords COVID-19, CARES Act, hospitals, safety net

As it has done for other dimensions of US society, the COVID-19 pandemic has exposed the vulnerability of our health care system and the enormous inequalities that exist within it. The US hospital system is marked by large and persistent inequalities. Health care in the United States has long been described as a "two-tier" health system in which patients with Medicare and private health insurance have access to a large number of hospitals,

Journal of Health Politics, Policy and Law, Vol. 46, No. 5, October 2021
DOI 10.1215/03616878-9155977 © 2021 by Duke University Press

while the uninsured and patients covered by Medicaid have access to a much smaller set of hospitals typically referred to as the health care safety net, which includes public hospitals, academic medical centers, and some community-based nonprofit hospitals (Davis and Schoen 1978; Stevens and Stevens 1974).

When the COVID-19 pandemic arrived in the United States, the entire hospital system suffered. When elective procedures were postponed during the first months of the pandemic, this resulted in significant revenue loss for all hospitals because they earn much higher payments from elective procedures than they do from emergency department admissions. Elective procedures account for about one-third of total inpatient hospital revenues. During the four-month period between March 1 and June 30, 2020, US hospitals and health systems lost more than $202 billion, or about $55 billion per month, because of a 40–45% decrease in operating revenue for the average hospital (AHA 2020).

In addition to a reduction in profitable procedures, many hospitals also suffered financially because they cared for a disproportionate share of patients with COVID-19. This is true, of course, because positive COVID-19 cases were not disbursed evenly throughout the country (or even within various states). The US health care system is bifurcated into what many have called "have" and "have-not" hospitals (Berenson 2015). Even after passage of the Affordable Care Act, government support for safety net and Medicaid policies that serve vulnerable populations is less generous and easier to cut than policies and programs that serve privately insured and Medicare patients (Allen et al. 2014; Grogan and Park 2017; Gusmano, Rodwin, and Weisz 2017; Soss, Fording, and Schram 2011). Because Black and Brown patients are more likely to be uninsured or Medicaid beneficiaries than white patients (Cohen, Martinez, and Zammitti 2016), and state Medicaid programs continue to pay substantially less than private insurance, this "racial payer gap"—along with racial residential segregation—continues to result in de facto racial segregation in the US hospital system (Blustein 2008; Caldwell et al. 2017; Chan et al. 2012; Hall and Rosenbaum 2012; Serwer 2009; Yang, Zhao, and Song 2017).

While the loss of revenue associated with the elimination of elective procedures is most applicable to wealthy hospitals, the "have-not" hospitals—those with poor financial performance prior to the onset of COVID-19—faced even more challenges because they disproportionately take care of low-income and uninsured patients, and patients from Black and Brown communities, who were disproportionately affected by COVID-19 (Garcia et al. 2021). Hospitals with a large share of COVID-19 patients experienced higher expenses owing to the need to acquire necessary equipment and supplies, and the higher labor costs associated with the surge in demand for hospital services and personnel (AHA 2020). As such, and unlike wealthier hospitals, the financial situation of safety net hospitals that had a large share of COVID-19 patients was made worse. In sum, all hospitals needed help but for different reasons.

The point of public policy is to decide which needs are most important and should take priority. This was the crucial question before Congress when members voted on the Coronavirus Aid, Relief, and Economic Security (CARES) Act, which was passed and signed into law by President Donald Trump on March 27, 2020. The CARES Act provided more than $2 trillion "to protect the American people from the public health and economic impacts of COVID-19."[1] Most of the legislation focused on relief to the general economy, particularly funding for the unemployed and small businesses; however, $175 billion was allocated to provide aid to the American health care system.

The purpose of this article is to first document how local policy elites, congressional members, and policy experts discussed what the intent of provider relief funding should be—which hospitals were considered most worthy of relief funding and why? Second, we examine how relief funds were actually distributed by the federal government to determine how the distribution matched various distributional arguments and congressional intent. We start by providing historical and recent evidence on inequities among hospitals in the United States. This provides a context to understand different arguments launched by stakeholders and policy makers about how relief funds should be distributed. We then detail our methodological approach and present our findings and conclusions.

Setting the Context: Long-Standing and Growing Inequities among US Hospitals

Several factors are fundamental to understanding inequalities in the US hospital system, in terms of the patients served, how hospitals are paid, and whether hospitals have access to financing for capital investments. The lack of a universal social insurance scheme explains why different payers pay different amounts for patients. However, the United States also has particular tax policies that allow bifurcated treatment among hospitals.

1. Coronavirus Aid, Relief, and Economic Security Act. Pub. L. No. 116–136, 134 Stat. 281 (2020).

In the 1960s state governments began to offer nonprofit hospitals more favorable lending conditions under the tax-exempt bond, which catapulted nonprofit hospitals into the capital credit markets. Debt financing increased from 38% of total financing for hospital construction in 1968 to 69% in 1981 (AHA 1986; Cohodes and Kinkead 1984). The dollar volume of health-care debt issues in the tax-exempt market went from $22 billion (5.7% of total issues) in 1974 to $75 billion (12.3%) in 1982. In just one year, from 1980 to 1981, hospitals and other health care institutions borrowed more than $5 billion in the long-term tax-exempt bond market. This represented a 40% increase from the 1980 level.

The increased reliance on private capital markets played a central role in creating a fundamental transformation toward the corporatization of the American health care system (Ermann and Gabel 1984; IOM 1983). The implications of this shift toward corporatization were threefold. First, reliance on private capital encouraged the formation of multihospital systems. The percent of US community hospitals affiliated with systems increased from 31% in 1979 to 53% in 2001 (Bazzoli 2004). Because large organizations could support the overhead necessary to develop sophisticated financial strategies, investment advisers and bond-rating agencies viewed multihospital systems as more financially stable (Brown and Saltman 1985). Because the credit rating of multi-institutional systems tended to be higher than single-facility hospitals, there was a strong motivation to join multihospital systems. For example, while 23% and 38% of multi-hospital systems had AA(+/-) and A+ ratings respectively, only 2% and 16% of single-facility hospitals had such ratings (IOM 1983). It is important to note that these mergers and acquisitions occurred regardless of ownership: nonprofit voluntary hospitals also experienced a growing number of corporate mergers and large-scale joint ventures (IOM 1983; Siegrist 1983).

Second, the shift toward reliance on private capital created explosive growth of proprietary hospital chains. The number of short-term acute care hospitals owned by for-profit hospital chains rose from 6% in 1977 to 10% in 1982. The five largest chains more than doubled their total beds during the same time period (Ermann and Gabel 1984; IOM 1983; Relman 1980). In 1990 33% of system hospitals were owned by for-profit systems (about one in four hospital beds) (Bazzoli 2004).

Third, the reliance on capital markets further bifurcated the US health care system. While public subsidies to access tax-exempt bonds were made easier for nonprofit hospitals in the post-1965 period, public hospitals were unable to take comparable advantage of subsidies attached to the tax-exempt bond markets. Because public hospitals had a higher proportion of

Medicaid patients among their payer mix, even private investors in the tax-exempt bond market with more lax rules saw them as a greater risk (Cleverley and Nutt 1984). This lower risk rating was clearly biased against a larger minority patient base and where many public hospitals were situated—in poorer minority neighborhoods in urban centers. While nonprofit hospitals serving predominantly white patients were welcomed into the capital markets, public hospitals (and other community hospitals with large Medicaid populations) were deemed a "bad risk" (Kinney and Lefkowitz 1982: 653).

Once they were deemed a bad risk, public hospitals found it very difficult to change their risk rating. Because public hospitals had much lower capital investment, their level of payments based on debt principal was low. As a result, it was difficult to build up an internal revenue base to use as leverage. Instead, public hospitals used a large portion of their discretionary funds to cover operating deficits, especially to meet the requirements of their mission to care for nonpaying patients. This stopgap measure led to future problems; since there was little capital investment, the amount of reimbursement continued to decline, and, as a result, discretionary funds continued to dwindle, and a downward cycle ensued. By the mid-1980s, several studies confirmed that public and nonprofit voluntary hospitals that served a disproportionate number of Black, Latino, and poor residents were much less likely to have access to capital markets than those hospitals that served predominately white residents with private insurance (Cleverley and Nutt 1984; Feder and Hadley 1983; Kinney and Lefkowitz 1982; Schatzkin 1984).

At the same time that states opened up the capital markets to nonprofit hospitals through the tax-exempt bond, in 1969 the IRS enacted a major change in interpreting charitable care for tax-exempt hospitals. As a result of the passage of Medicare and Medicaid, the IRS accepted the American Hospital Association's claim that "they couldn't find patients to whom to give free care" (Fox and Schaffer 1991). As part of its 1969 ruling, the IRS applied a far broader definition of "charitable" to hospitals wherein "the promotion of health is considered to be a charitable purpose" (Fox and Schaffer 1991). The IRS concluded that a hospital could be tax-exempt "even though the class of beneficiaries eligible to receive a direct benefit from its activities does not include . . . indigent members of the community."[2] This IRS ruling legally allowed nonprofit hospitals access to state-subsidized capital

---

2. Coronavirus Aid, Relief, and Economic Security Act. Pub. L. No. 116–136, 134 Stat. 281 (2020).

markets to invest in hospital renovations and new technology to distinguish themselves (as much as they could) as hospitals for the middle and upper class (by primarily accepting those with private insurance and Medicare) while leaving (and in many cases pushing) the poor and uninsured on to public hospitals.

While all nonprofit hospitals enjoy tax exempt status and can technically take advantage of the 1969 IRS ruling, not all do. Many small community-based nonprofit hospitals—especially those located in communities with high poverty rates and a high proportion of residents of color, or in rural areas—maintain a mission that predominantly serves the un- and under-insured and Medicaid beneficiaries. Like public hospitals, these non-profit community-based hospitals have difficulty accessing the capital markets and taking advantage of tax-exempt bonds. Thus, over time, a strict demarcation emerged between the "have-not" safety net hospitals, which include public and some nonprofit hospitals, and the "have" hospitals, which include for-profit and some nonprofit hospitals with access to capital markets.

Despite enormous subsidies to the health care system—funding at least 70% of total national health expenditures (Pauly 2019)—the government's role in planning the health care system is largely restricted to antitrust rulings in the courts, and those decisions have largely turned in favor of mergers and acquisitions in the last three decades (Capps et al. 2019). While the number of multihospital systems increased from the 1970s to 2000, the growth in health system consolidations since 2000 has been enormous. Between 1998 and 2015, there were 1,410 hospital mergers and acquisitions in the United States (Pope 2019). By 2010, the top five hospitals or systems accounted for 88% of market power (Cutler and Morton 2013). Since 2010 average annual hospital merger volume has surged by 50% compared to the prior decade (Kaufman Hall 2018), and by 2018 "91 percent of hospital beds were in system-affiliated hospitals—an increase from 88 percent in 2016" (Furukawa et al. 2020). As consolidation has increased significantly, there is growing evidence that hospital and provider organizations have garnered monopoly-like power and are able to command significantly higher prices from commercial insurers (Cooper et al. 2019; Ginsburg and Pawlson 2014; MedPAC 2020). The main way hospitals are profitable is to charge high prices to private insurance, which is why they prefer privately insured patients over publicly insured patients (Ly and Cutler 2018).

Health system consolidations since 2010 have exacerbated hospital inequities. There are now not just "have" but "must-have" hospitals that are able to obtain among the highest rates of payments from commercial payers, often exceeding 250% of Medicare's allowed payment (Berenson 2015). In a study of 13 health care markets, there was evidence of a wide gap between the highest- and lowest-priced hospitals; in three markets, the highest-priced hospital was paid well above twice as much as the lowest-priced hospital for inpatient services (White, Bond, and Reschovsky 2013). And, with these high prices, as Robert Berenson (2015: 713) explains, "these prestigious organizations are able to set aside huge reserves and compensate their executives quite generously." As such, the wealthy health systems with monopoly-like power have contributed significantly not only to the enormous health care expenditure problem in the United States but also to further bifurcation in the system (Berenson 2015; Rosenthal 2019). Of course, as the data above attest, many of these large, consolidated health care systems were quite wealthy before the pandemic hit. The median US hospital had more than 53 days of cash on hand, but some of the largest and wealthiest not-for-profit hospital systems had two to three times that amount of cash on hand (Liss 2020). Moody's Investors Service rated the bonds of 284 hospitals in 2018, and 50% had enough cash on hand to cover at least six months of operating costs with no revenues (Rau 2020). In contrast, the poorest 25% of all hospitals in the United States (including public, non-profit, and for-profit hospitals) had only enough cash on hand to pay for a week (7.6 days) of their operating expenses (Khullar, Bond, and Schpero 2020).

When the pandemic hit, it was quite clear that some hospitals—certainly those with more than 100 days of cash on hand—would be well equipped financially to withstand the COVID-19 storm, while others in a more financially volatile position would not be equipped. Thus it is not surprising that when provider relief funds were forthcoming early in the pandemic, there was concern about how different hospitals would be treated and whether greater financial vulnerability would be taken into account. Before summarizing the main distributional arguments for hospital relief payments, we turn first to describing our methods.

Methods

A two-pronged methodological approach was used to determine congressional intent and common arguments launched for how provider relief funds should be distributed, and how the actual distribution matched these intentions and arguments. To determine congressional and stakeholder intentions for how provider relief funds should be used, we reviewed

Table 1 Provider Relief Fund Distributions, Target, and Funding

Distribution	Timing	Target/formula	Total funds
1st general fund	April 10 and 24	Medicare FFS providers/ net patient revenue	$50 billion
2nd rural providers	May 6	Rural acute hospitals and critical access hospitals	$10 billion
3rd high impact	May 7	Hospitals with at least 100 COVID-19 admissions	$12 billion
4th safety net hospitals	June 9	Hospitals with large number of Medicaid and uninsured patients	$10.2 billion

Note: There were other smaller distributions, such as $7.4 billion to nursing homes; however, in this analysis, we focused on the distribution of funding to hospitals. The rural distribution also included rural health clinics and community health centers, but we focused on rural hospitals.
Source: Congressional Research Service 2020.

several documents and policy discourse at the local and federal levels. The legislation itself clearly stated the intention of the relief funds; however, letters from members of Congress to the secretary of the Department of Health and Human Services (HHS) after the release of some provider relief funds also provide some evidence of bipartisan agreement as to how funds should be distributed. Moreover, media stories with key stakeholders, expert reports, and opinion pieces provide additional evidence of common concerns about the distribution of funds.

Second, to examine how provider relief funds (PRF) were actually distributed, we use data from HHS (n.d.). The provider relief funds were allocated to hospitals according to four distributional schemes: general, high-impact, rural, and safety net (see table 1). The first allocation—the "general" distribution—allocated $50 billion and focused on reimbursing hospitals based on concerns about revenues lost, whereas the "high-impact" (also called the hot-spot) distribution allocated $12 billion and focused on COVID-19 need. The remaining two distributions targeted allocations to hospitals in financial distress according to their location in rural areas or designation as a safety net provider.

The PRF data report provides name, state, city, and payment amount for the first $50 billion general distribution and the $12 billion high-impact distribution. They also report the amount of funding allocated to each state, and the number of providers receiving funding in each state, for both the rural and safety net distributions. Based on this more detailed information, we calculate more fine-tuned estimates for these distributions using the formulas and comparing back to the state-level data (for exact formulas, see appendix A in the online appendix).

By September 2020, 4,674 hospitals had received some amount of provider relief funding. Hospitals did not have to apply for aid. If a hospital met the distributional requirement, it was sent a payment. Almost all hospitals that received funding accepted and attested to receiving it.

To examine how funds were allocated to particular types of hospitals, we utilize data from the most recent Medicare Cost Reports (2018) accessed from the RAND Corporation Healthcare Provider Cost Reporting Information System (HCRIS) files. Based on our policy and media review, which will be presented in the findings section below, three main distributional arguments emerged. To determine if the PRF payments were allocated according to these distributional arguments, we identify a measurement strategy for each. Here we briefly describe each distributional argument (though more detail as to where the argument comes from is provided in the findings section below) and the associated measurement.

The first main distributional argument was to provide relief to hospitals that suffered from revenue losses as a result of the elimination of elective procedures during COVID-19. Although there is no data that separates elective from nonelective procedures, most surgeries and outpatient procedures were eliminated during this time period and could therefore be used as a proxy for revenue loss. In particular, because hospitals vary substantially in the extent to which they rely on surgical and outpatient revenue streams, some hospitals will experience more revenue loss because of COVID-19 restrictions (Khullar, Bond, and Schpero 2020). We used the RAND dataset to calculate the percentage of total revenue from outpatient services.

The second main distributional argument claimed that hospitals with high financial vulnerability should receive relief funds. One measure to capture financial vulnerability is days cash on hand. This is a common measure of an organization's level of cash resources. It is an estimate of the number of days an organization could operate if no cash were collected or received. The exact measure is [Cash + Temporary Investments + Investments]/ [(Total expenses - Depreciation)/Days in period]. This is a particularly good measure to determine if a hospital is able to get through a crisis like COVID-19, which represented a significant cash flow crunch. For example, if a hospital has 90–180 days cash on hand, it can operate for 3 to 6 months without any additional revenue. In contrast, those hospitals with fewer than seven days cash on hand have a week or less to operate without any additional revenue. To get through the COVID-19 cash crunch, those hospitals would have had to borrow money, sell assets, or seek emergency funding. Without assistance, the hospital would fail to meet its next payroll (NCRHRP 2020).

Although there are other measures of financial performance, such as operating margin, current asset-to-liability ratio, and days in net accounts receivable (Khullar, Bond, and Schpero 2020), these measures are better for reflecting longer-term financial performance. Because the PRFs were distributed for the very purpose of temporary crisis assistance, days cash on hand is the best measure to determine if hospitals most in crisis of not being able to meet their daily operating expenses were provided assistance on par with hospitals that had more secure cash reserves.

For days cash on hand, and percent outpatient revenues, we calculate tertiles to illustrate how hospitals with low, medium, and high levels of days cash on hand and percent outpatient revenues receive significantly different average provider relief payments per bed.

The third distributional argument suggested that the PRFs should address both financial vulnerability and revenue losses. Because each of the four distributions was created by HHS to address these different concerns, we analyze the total allocation to hospitals across all four distributions to determine whether both concerns—financial vulnerability and revenues lost—were treated equally in the allocation of relief funding.

We conduct a multivariate regression to determine if these two main variables—days cash on hand and outpatient share of revenues—are significant when controlling for other hospital characteristics that might also impact the distribution of PRF payments. We control for the following hospital characteristics, which are often associated with financial performance: health system membership, ownership, teaching status, "critical access" hospital status, and occupancy rate. We do not control for the factors that HHS used to determine the PRF distributions, notably COVID-19 need, rural, safety net, and net revenues, because they would essentially explain all the variation. We are interested instead in understanding the substantive implications of using distributional formulas based on these factors.

A few other studies analyze provider relief payments by hospital characteristics (Khullar, Bond, and Schpero 2020; Schwartz and Damico 2020). In general, their findings suggest, based on HHS's formula for the first distribution, that hospitals with higher financial performance would receive higher PRF payments. While these were important early findings, they did not account for the three other distributions that HHS claimed would award payments to the more financially vulnerable hospitals. Our study examines actual PRF payments for the first two distributions (not simulations of the formulas) and analyzes payments across all four distributions to determine which distributional arguments were privileged when and how.

Finally, as discussed below, another voiced concern was that the PRFs should be distributed to hospitals that serve a disproportionate number of Black and Brown patients. Unfortunately, the RAND dataset does not include patient demographic information by hospital. Searching other hospital datasets, such as data from the American Hospital Association, we could find no information on patient race by hospital. Pragya Kakani and colleagues (2020) analyze relief funding and race, but they look at counties as the unit of analysis. Many use safety net hospitals as a proxy for race because it is known that a disproportionate number of Black and Brown patients access safety net hospitals for inpatient care. This is imperfect because patient racial demographics vary widely across safety net hospitals.

Findings

Stakeholder Arguments and Congressional Intent

By the time the pandemic visibly arrived in March 2020, the reality of a separate and unequal hospital system, in which poor people will be treated in poor institutions, was largely accepted without question. Many were outraged when the early reports of huge racial disparities in COVID-19 deaths were announced, but that did not translate into dramatic (or even small) changes in how the health care system responded or in the public discourse about how the system should respond. Instead, public discourse focused on the need to provide assistance to address COVID-19–related racial disparities. Public discourse around racial disparities and COVID-19 in Chicago helps illustrate discourse at the local level.

On April 6, 2020, the Chicago public health department had just released data showing that while Black residents made up 30% of Chicago's population, they accounted for 52% of the city's lab-confirmed cases of COVID-19 and 72% of Chicago's deaths. In response, Chicago's Mayor Lori E. Lightfoot said, "Those numbers take your breath away. It's unacceptable. No one should think this is OK." That same night, Carol Marin, a reporter from a local news program, *Chicago Tonight*, asked health care administrator Sean O'Grady, from North Shore University Health System, about the degree to which his system, and other hospitals with greater financial capacity, were helping to support safety net hospitals in Chicago.

Mr. O'Grady, safety net hospitals on the West and the South sides [of Chicago] are in more serious need of equipment versus more affluent hospitals, not unlike North Shore, is there a sharing at all going on *between the more affluent with the less affluent*?

In response, Mr. O'Grady said,

Well, Carol, as you know, Swedish Covenant Hospital joined North Shore earlier this year and we have been working very closely with them as a safety net hospital that's a part of our system to ensure that they have the appropriate supplies and equipment that they need. And, that they are taken care of just as we are taking care of our folks in the Legacy North Shore System.

Carol Martin continued to press him on the extent to which "more affluent" hospitals were helping safety net hospitals, even if they were not part of the same hospital system. She asked,

But, *hospitals in a classic sense compete against each other*, [however] in this plague it's a different sort of story. So, what is the kind of sharing that might be happening or is it not?

Rather than address the issue directly, Mr. O'Grady shifted to a discussion of how the state was working to bring providers together.

So, I talk to my colleagues around the city on a regular basis, to find out what they're doing in various domains of the response plans and we are regularly talking about how we can help one another . . . uhm, I know my colleagues and I are very committed to sharing across the market. (Caine 2020)

This exchange illustrates how hospital inequalities are normalized by both speakers. Neither raised questions about whether there should be such an enormous financial disparity among the hospitals treating residents of Chicago; it was accepted as an immutable fact of reality. On a television news program, the terms *more affluent* and *less affluent* are used to describe the health care system as normal, and the question is how—or whether—the less affluent should be helped during this crisis, and voluntary "sharing between affluent and less affluent" is left intentionally vague.

On the same day that the public health department announced the high rates of COVID-19 among Black and Brown Chicagoans, the public hospital system, Stroger Health System, announced it would temporarily close Provident Hospital's emergency room—located in a community that is

95% Black with a third of the population living below the poverty level. In response to the closure, the president of the Chicago Medical Society, Dr. Jay Chauhan, said, "In the safety net hospitals—those hospitals with a lower degree of resources in more fiscally challenged areas—they are having more trouble . . . whereas some larger [more affluent health networks are well-resourced, and] were able to prepare for this in a more timely fashion." Dr. Chauhan's comments highlight the existence of a two-tiered hospital system in the United States, and he suggests, on behalf of the Chicago Medical Society, that hospitals with high financial vulnerability in "fiscally challenged areas" should receive more assistance during the COVID-19 crisis.

When the federal government passed the CARES Act and provided $175 billion for hospitals and physicians, the expressed intent of the Provider Relief Funds was, as written in the legislation, "to reimburse, through grants or other mechanisms, eligible health care providers for health care related expenses or lost revenues that are attributable to coronavirus."[3] Although not very detailed, the legislation clearly incorporates a distributional argument—that PRFs should be distributed to alleviate hospitals' financial stress caused by expenses of responding to COVID-19 need and lost revenue because of COVID-19 restrictions.

Many questions about fairness were raised based on the timing, allocation determinations, and funding amounts for these various distributions. First, because the funding amount to hospitals for the first allocation was based on net patient revenues, there was concern that HHS was prioritizing potential revenues lost during the COVID-19 pandemic over those hospitals that took on a disproportionate amount of COVID-19 patients. We emphasize "potential" revenues lost because at the time of disbursement it was not clear which hospitals would ultimately, at the end of the year, experience net revenue loss or gains. Second, and relatedly, because the first allocation was based on net patient revenues, the allocation may have rewarded hospitals in better financial health, not necessarily those hospitals that experienced the most financial harm—especially in the long-term. Third, although the high-impact allocation focused on hospitals with high COVID-19 need, these hospitals had to wait for payments, which were distributed a month after the first release of funding (May 7 compared to April 10). Fourth, the total funding amounts were lower for the high-impact distribution ($12 billion) compared to the first general distribution ($50 billion), which raised concerns about whether hospitals that took on a

---

3. Pub. L. No. 116–136 (March 27, 2020), section 3203, subpart B.

disproportionate number of COVID-19 patients would be adequately compensated. Finally, there was concern that safety net hospitals would have to wait much too long to receive financial help, given that many safety net hospitals in major US cities were on the front lines of the pandemic.

On May 7, 2020, Representative Frank Pallone Jr. (D-NJ), chair of the House Committee on Energy and Commerce, and Representative Richard Neal (D-MA), chair of the Committee on Ways and Means, sent a joint letter to Alex Azar, the secretary of Health and Human Services, and Seema Verma, the administrator of the Centers for Medicare and Medicaid Services (CMS). The two committee chairs raised several concerns about the HHS hospital allocation formula. First, they raised concern about "the lack of transparency with Congress and the American people about how funds are being spent or loans are being made . . . [and] who has received funds," and requested that all of the data on all distributions from the Provider Relief Fund be provided to Congress without further delay. Second, they argued that the formula used for the general fund was flawed because it was not targeted to providers in greatest need. As they put it, "The approach adopted clearly fails to target funding based on the statutory framework relating to COVID-19 driven costs, and in fact the level of funding appears to be completely disconnected from need" (Pallone and Neal 2020).

Less than one month after chairmen Pallone and Neal wrote their letter, Senator Charles Grassley (R-IA), the chair of the Senate Finance Committee; Senator Ron Wyden (D-OR), the ranking member on the Senate Finance Committee; Representative Pallone; and Representative Greg Walden (R-OR), the ranking member on the House Energy and Commerce Committee wrote another letter to Secretary Azar raising specific concerns about the failure of the department to allocate funds to Medicaid providers. This bipartisan group wrote:

> As the chairs and ranking members of the committees of jurisdiction over the Medicaid program, we are concerned that the delay in disbursing funds from the Public Health and Social Services Emergency Fund (PHSSEF) for Medicaid-dependent providers could result in long term financial hardship for providers who serve some of our most vulnerable populations. It could also severely hamper their ability to continue to serve as essential providers amid the COVID-19 pandemic and beyond. (Grassley et al. 2020)

As with the previous letter from Pallone and Neal, this letter raised concerns about the HHS formula and argued that the department was delaying payments to providers in greatest need. The letter stated: "HHS has, thus far, relied on methodologies that favor providers that receive a larger share of their payments from Medicare or private insurance" (Grassley, Wyden, and Walden 2020). In the context of a politically polarized Congress, this show of bipartisan concern about how HHS allocated the CARES Act funds is noteworthy.

Multiple reports and industry publications also raised concern about the allocation of funds. On April 27 the *Washington Post* published an article with the headline, "Amid Coronavirus Distress, Wealthy Hospitals Hoard Millions," in which it documented how safety net hospitals with little cash on hand were competing with wealthy hospitals for federal relief funds (Rau 2020). On May 26 articles in the *New York Times* and *Becker's Healthcare*, an influential industry publication, noted that the 20 largest hospital systems received $5 billion in government funds, even though these systems were holding more than $100 billion in reserves (Drucker, Silver-Greenberg, and Kliff 2020; Ellison 2020).

Based on local and national policy discourse, CARES legislation, and publications critiquing how PRFs were distributed, three main distributional arguments emerge. First, the hospital industry lobbied for relief funding to address the problem of lost revenue as a result of COVID-19 restrictions. The first general distribution developed by HHS addressed this concern. The formula relied primarily on net patient revenues from 2018 to determine PRF payments to hospitals in this first allocation of $50 billion. As discussed above, many immediately raised concerns that this formula would disproportionately reward hospitals in good financial condition, and was not adequately tied to revenues lost because of COVID-19 restrictions. As discussed in the methods section, we analyze the percent of outpatient revenues to determine whether hospitals with a higher share of outpatient revenues received more PRF payments on average.

A second concern expressed early at the local level, and in response to HHS's formula for the general distribution, argued that the PRF allocation should be based on financial vulnerability and the extent to which hospitals could operate during the COVID-19 crisis. We analyze days cash on hand to determine whether hospitals with low cash reserves received more on average PRF payments as one would hope under the logic of this distributional argument.

Finally, the third distributional argument, embedded in the legislative language, suggested that the PRF payments should balance these competing concerns. Indeed, the four distributions did each attempt to address these different distributional arguments: 1) general distribution addressed revenue lost, 2) high-impact distribution addressed COVID-19 need, 3) the safety net, and 4) rural distributions addressed concerns about financially vulnerable hospitals. Yet because the amount of funding for each distribution varied, it raised the question—does combined funding across all four distributions equally balance these competing concerns?

How Does the Actual Distribution of Funds Match the Distributional Arguments?

Although we use graphs to illustrate the bivariate relationships of interest below, all reported significance levels are based on multivariate regression analyses controlling for variables listed in the methods section. The models are all significant according to F-tests, and the control variables are all significant in the expected direction (appendix B in the online appendix).

Revenues Lost. The purpose of the general distribution was to provide relief to hospitals that experienced major revenue losses as a result of the elimination of elective procedures during COVID-19 restrictions. Using the outpatient share of a hospital's total revenue, it is clear that hospitals with the highest potential revenue losses were provided substantially more relief funding than those with lower levels of reliance on elective procedures for revenues (see fig. 1). Those hospitals with more than 80% of their revenue coming from outpatient procedures received about $97,000 per bed on average compared to $26,488 per bed for hospitals with less than 60% outpatient revenue share. As one would expect, the relationship was reversed for the high-impact distribution based on COVID-19 need. Those hospitals that rely heavily on outpatient revenues (i.e., elective procedures) received only $432 per bed on average compared to those hospitals with the lowest share of outpatient revenues—about $18,000 per bed on average.

Financial Vulnerability. The safety net and rural distributions were specifically aimed at hospitals that suffer more financial vulnerability during the COVID-19 crisis, and especially in terms of safety net hospitals, take care of a disproportionate amount of Medicaid and uninsured patients. Although all hospitals that met these definitions benefitted from relief payments, the allocation did not disproportionately help the most financially vulnerable within these groups (see fig. 2). Safety net hospitals with more than 76 days of cash on hand received about the same average PRF payments per bed as those with fewer than 3 days cash on hand. Among rural hospitals, those with more than 76 days cash on hand received almost $8,000 per bed on average compared to $4,500 per bed for those rural hospitals with fewer than 3 days cash on hand.

Interestingly, the high-impact distribution awarded higher average PRF payments to more financially vulnerable hospitals. Because this distribution

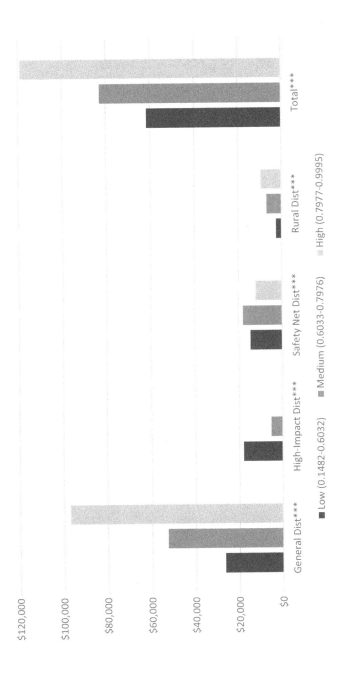

Figure 1 Average provider relief fund payment per bed by outpatient share of revenue.

Note: *** = <= 0.001 significance level is based on OLS regression results as described in the Methods section above and provided in appendix B of the online-only appendix.

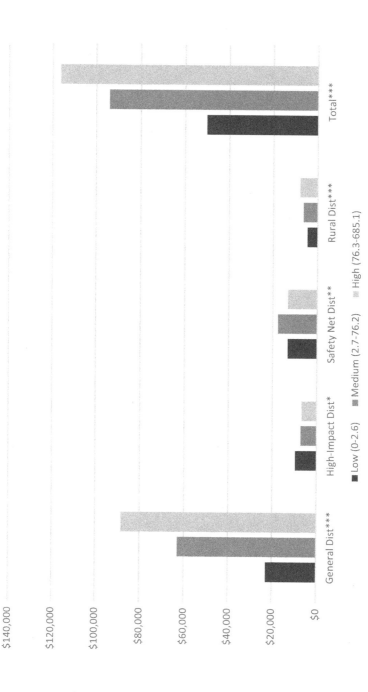

Figure 2 Average provider relief fund payment per bed by days of cash on hand.

Note: * = <0.05, ** = <0.01, and *** = <=0.001 significance levels are based on OLS regression results as described in the Methods section above and provided in appendix B of the online-only appendix.

was based on the number of COVID-19 cases over 100 in each hospital, it is clear that hospitals with less cash on hand experienced higher COVID-19 impact. In particular, among hospitals with high COVID-19 impact, those with fewer than 3 days cash on hand received $9,637 per bed payments on average compared to $6,737 per bed for hospitals with more than 76 days cash on hand.

Finally, although the general distribution was intended to provide relief to hospitals with high revenue loss, figure 2 makes starkly clear how this formula also disproportionately rewarded hospitals with more financial security. Hospitals that could operate without assistance for more than two months (76 days cash on hand) during the COVID-19 crisis received $88,000 per bed on average compared to $23,000 per bed on average for hospitals with less than a week of cash on hand.

Balance Competing Concerns: Revenue Loss, COVID-19 Impact and Financial Vulnerability? Although it is clear that hospitals with better financial performance were the first to receive relief payments, and they received higher average payments per bed from that first general distribution, an important question is whether the overall payments evened out over time after HHS was able to provide the additional distributions based on COVID-19 need and hospital financial vulnerability—rural location and safety net status. To analyze this question, we calculated total payments across all four distributions (see "Total" columns in figs. 1 and 2). Overall, the four distributions from the CARES Act allocated substantially higher average relief payments per bed to hospitals with potential revenue loss associated with the elimination of outpatient procedures, and to hospitals with higher levels of financial security (more than 76 days cash on hand).

Conclusion: COVID-19 Relief Funds Fuel Hospital Inequities

We began this inquiry by noting that the US hospital system is marked by large and persistent inequalities. It is a two-tier health system in which hospitals with high financial performance tend to take care of patients with Medicare and private health insurance and predominantly white patients, whereas hospitals with low financial performance tend to take care of the uninsured and patients covered by Medicaid and predominantly Black and Brown patients.

The United States could have responded to hospital vulnerability during the COVID-19 crisis when it was clear that Black and Brown patients were suffering disproportionately from COVID-19 by providing higher-on-average relief payments to financially vulnerable hospitals. Instead, it did

the opposite. It privileged concerns about revenue loss over other articulated concerns, and those hospitals with the most financial security received
the most relief. Thus, at a time when racial inequities were on stark display, the United States chose to allocate funding in ways that continued to
fuel these inequities (see Fink 2021 for a recent investigative report of this
situation in Los Angeles).

One might argue—as many actually did—that providing relief to all
hospitals including the more financially well-off is important because of
their impact on local economies. Yet, while public officials hoped relief
funds might prevent layoffs and furloughs, the only requirement put in place
for the receipt of COVID-19 provider funds was to not charge uninsured
COVID-19 patients (since hospitals would be reimbursed separately) and
to agree to no "surprise (out-of-network) billing" for COVID-19 patients.
The lack of any stipulations meant that many hospitals receiving payments
still furloughed workers.

Moreover, even if one might agree that multiple reasons for financial
hardship—lost revenue, COVID-19 need, and financial vulnerability—are
worthy, there is no logical reason that average payments for one reason
(revenues lost) should substantially outweigh the other (COVID-19 need).
In this sense, the allocation of CARES Act funds reflects perhaps the most
profound aspects of political power. The administration rewarded those
hospitals that cater to the most privileged in the United States, leaving
hospitals that predominantly serve low-income people of color with less.
In terms of distributional equity, the allocation of Provider Relief Funds to
address the COVID-19 crisis can only bluntly be described as unsanitized
and unfair.

These findings also reveal how structural inequities and structural racism
are embedded in the organization and financing of the US hospital system.
As long as the United States continues to rely on a two-tiered health care
financing system with significantly lower payments to hospitals that care for
a high proportion of indigent patients and Black and Brown patients, policies
that address short-term financial crises, like the one caused by the pandemic,
will likely replicate this pattern. Specifically, distributional policies that rely
on "revenues lost" and broad definitions of "safety net" hospitals without
explicitly considering the implications of the allocation of funding by race
and its impact on poor and Black and Brown communities will further
embed—and hide—policies that enhance race and income inequalities.

To begin to undo this pattern of structural racism within the hospital
system, the federal government should require all Medicare-participating
hospitals to submit aggregate data on the racial composition of all their

patients. This would allow for much greater transparency in racial variations in policies and treatment across US hospitals. However, more important would be to address the root cause of structural racism and inequity across hospitals. Future health reform in the United States should focus not only on expanding insurance coverage but also on creating a more uniform national system of payments. Doing so would not only simplify the administration of the health care system and provide the government with a tool for reducing health care inflation (Gusmano et al. 2020), it would also eliminate one of the factors that created and continues to reinforce a bifurcated hospital system.

■ ■ ■

Colleen M. Grogan is a professor at the University of Chicago's Crown Family School. Her research interests include the role of private provision in health policy, the structure of public entitlements, and implications for health equity. She received an NIH-funded book grant titled *The Rise of the Conservative Health Care State*. She has a new coauthored project on the role of private equity in health care and several NIH-funded collaborative projects focused on the impact of Medicaid policies on access to substance use disorder treatment. She is co-associate editor of health policy for the *American Journal of Public Health*.
cgrogan@uchicago.edu

Michael K. Gusmano is a professor with the School of Public Health's Department of Health Behavior, Society, and Policy and Administration at Rutgers University. He also is a research scholar at the Hastings Center and a visiting fellow at the Nelson A. Rockefeller Institute of Government of the State University of New York. He serves as the international editor of the *Journal of Aging and Social Policy*; is an associate editor for *Health Economics, Policy and Law*; is on the board of editors of the *Journal of Health Politics, Policy and Law*; and is on the editorial committee of the *Hastings Center Report*.

Yu-An Lin is an assistant professor with the Department of Social Work, National Taipei University, New Taipei City, Taiwan.

Acknowledgments

The authors thank the guest editors of *JHPPL* and two anonymous reviewers for their very helpful comments on an earlier version of this manuscript. We also acknowledge insightful feedback from workshop participants at the Michael Davis Seminar Series at the Center for Health Administration Studies, Crown Family School, University of Chicago.

References

AHA (American Hospital Association). 1986. "Survey of Sources of Funding for Hospital Construction," 1968, 1981. *Journal of Hospital Capital Finance,* no. 1: 8.

AHA (American Hospital Association). 2020. "Hospitals and Health Systems Face Unprecedented Financial Pressures Due to COVID-19." May 5. www.aha.org /guidesreports/2020-05-05-hospitals-and-health-systems-face-unprecedented -financial-pressures-due.

Allen, Heidi, Bill J. Wright, Kristin Harding, and Lauren Broffman. 2014. "The Role of Stigma in Access to Health Care for the Poor." *Milbank Quarterly* 92, no. 22: 289–318. doi.org/10.1111/1468-0009.12059.

Bazzoli, Gloria J. 2004. "The Corporatization of American Hospitals." *Journal of Health Politics, Policy and Law* 29, nos. 4–5: 885–905. doi.org/10.1215/03616878- 29-4-5-885.

Berenson, Robert. 2015. "Addressing Pricing Power in Integrated Delivery: The Limits of Antitrust." *Journal of Health Politics, Policy and Law* 40, no. 4: 711–44. doi.org/10.1215/03616878-3150026.

Blustein, Jan. 2008. "Who Is Accountable for Racial Equity in Health Care?" *JAMA* 299, no. 7: 814–16. doi.org/10.1001/jama.299.7.814.

Brown, Jonathan Betz, and Richard B. Saltman. 1985. "Health Capital Policy in the United States: A Strategic Perspective." *Inquiry* 22, no. 2: 122–31.

Caine, Paul. 2020. "Illinois Hospitals Strained but Largely Coping Ahead of Antici- pated COVID-19 Surge." WTTW News, April 6. news.wttw.com/2020/04/06 /illinois-hospitals-strained-largely-coping-ahead-anticipated-covid-19-surge.

Caldwell, Julia T., Chandra L. Ford, Steven P. Wallace, May C. Wang, and Lois M. Takahashi. 2017. "Racial and Ethnic Residential Segregation and Access to Health Care in Rural Areas." *Health and Place* 43: 104–12. doi.org/10.1016/j.healthplace .2016.11.015.

Capps, Cory, Laura Kmitch, Zenon Zabinski, and Slava Zayats. 2019. "The Con- tinuing Saga of Hospital Merger Enforcement." *Antitrust Law Journal* 82, no. 2: 441–96.

Chan, Kitty S., Darrell J. Gaskin, Gniesha Y. Dinwiddie, and Rachael McCleary. 2012. "Do Diabetic Patients Living in Racially Segregated Neighborhoods Experience Different Access and Quality of Care?" *Medical Care* 50, no. 8: 692–99. doi.org/ 10.1097/MLR.0b013e318254a43c.

Cleverley, William O., and Paul C. Nutt. 1984. "The Decision Process Used for Hospital Bond Rating—and Its Implications." *Health Services Research* 19, no. 5: 615–37.

Cohen, Robin A., Michael E. Martinez, and Emily P. Zammitti. 2016. "Health Insurance Coverage: Early Release of Estimates from the National Health Inter- view Survey, 2015." National Health Interview Survey Early Release Program, May. www.cdc.gov/nchs/data/nhis/earlyrelease/insur201605.pdf.

Cohodes, Donald R., and Brian M. Kinkead. 1984. *Hospital Capital Formation in the 1980s.* Baltimore, MD: Johns Hopkins University Press.

Cooper, Zack, Stuart V. Craig, Martin Gaynor, and John Van Reenen. 2019. "The Price Ain't Right? Hospital Prices and Health Spending on the Privately Insured." *Quarterly Journal of Economics* 134, no. 1: 51–107. doi.org/10.1093/qje/qjy020.

Cutler, David M., and Fiona Scott Morton. 2013. "Hospitals, Market Share, and Consolidation." *JAMA* 310, no. 18: 1964–70. doi.org/10.1001/jama.2013.281675.

Davis, Karen, and Cathy Schoen. 1978. *Health and the War on Poverty: A Ten-Year Appraisal*. Washington, DC: Brookings Institution.

Drucker, Jesse, Jessica Silver-Greenberg, and Sarah Kliff. 2020. "Wealthiest Hospitals Got Billions in Bailout for Struggling Health Providers." *New York Times*, May 25.

Ellison, Ayla. 2020. "Forty-Two Hospitals Closed, Filed for Bankruptcy This Year." *Becker's Hospital CFO Report*, June 22. www.beckershospitalreview.com/finance /42-hospitals-closed-filed-for-bankruptcy-this-year.html.

Ermann, Dan, and Jon Gabel. 1984. "Multihospital Systems: Issues and Empirical Findings." *Health Affairs* 3, no. 1: 50–64. doi.org/10.1377/hlthaff.3.1.50.

Feder, Judith M., and Jack Hadley. 1983. *Cutbacks, Recession, and Care to the Poor: Will the Urban Poor Get Hospital Care?* Washington, DC: Urban Institute.

Fink, Sheri. 2021. "Dying of Covid in a 'Separate and Unequal' L.A. Hospital." *New York Times*, February 8. www.nytimes.com/2021/02/08/us/covid-los-angeles.html.

Fox, Daniel M., and Daniel C. Schaffer. 1991. "Tax Administration as Health Policy: The Tax Exemption of Hospitals, 1969–1990." *Tax Notes*, October 21.

Furukawa, Michael F., Laura Kimmey, David J. Jones, Rachel M. Machta, Jing Guo, and Eugene C. Rich. 2020. "Consolidation of Providers into Health Systems Increased Substantially, 2016–18." *Health Affairs* 39, no. 8: 1321–25. doi.org/10.1377/hlthaff .2020.00017.

Garcia, Marc A., Patricia A. Homan, Catherine García, and Tyson H. Brown. 2021. "The Color of COVID-19: Structural Racism and the Disproportionate Impact of the Pandemic on Older Black and Latinx Adults." *Journal of Gerontology: Series B* 76, no. 3: e75–e80. doi.org/10.1093/geronb/gbaa114.

Ginsburg, Paul B., and L. Gregory Pawlson. 2014. "Seeking Lower Prices Where Providers Are Consolidated: An Examination of Market and Policy Strategies." *Health Affairs* 3, no. 6: 1067–75. doi.org/10.1377/hlthaff.2013.0810.

Grassley, Charles E., Frank Pallone Jr., Ron Wyden, and Greg Walden. 2020. Letter to HHS Secretary Alex Azar. June 3. www.finance.senate.gov/imo/media/doc/060320% 20Medicaid%20Provider%20Fund%20Letter.pdf.

Grogan, Colleen M., and Sunggeun Ethan Park. 2017. "The Politics of Medicaid: Most Americans Are Connected to the Program, Support Its Expansion, and Do Not View It as Stigmatizing." *Milbank Quarterly* 95, no. 4: 749–82. doi.org/10.1111/1468-0009.12298.

Gusmano, Michael K., Miriam Laugesen, Lawrence D. Brown, and Victor G. Rodwin. 2020. "Getting the Price Right: What Other Countries Do Well." *Health Affairs* 39, no. 11. doi.org/10.1377/hlthaff.2019.01804.

Gusmano, Michael K., Victor G. Rodwin, and Daniel Weisz. 2017. "Persistent Inequalities in Health and Access to Health Services: Evidence from New York City." *World Medical and Health Policy* 9, no. 2: 186–205.

Hall, Mark A., and Sara Rosenbaum. 2012. *The Health Care Safety Net in a Post-Reform World*. New Brunswick, NJ: Rutgers University Press.

HHS (US Department of Health and Human Services). n.d. "CARES Act Provider Relief Fund: Data." www.hhs.gov/coronavirus/cares-act-provider-relief-fund/data /index.html?language=en (accessed April 12, 2021).

IOM (Institute of Medicine). 1983. *The New Health Care for Profit: Doctors and Hospitals in a Competitive Environment*, edited by Bradford H. Gray. Washington, DC: National Academies Press.

Kakani, Pragya, Amitabh Chandra, Sendhil Mullainathan, and Ziad Obermeyer. 2020. "Allocation of COVID-19 Relief Funding to Disproportionately Black Counties." *JAMA* 324, no. 10: 1000–1003. doi.org/10.1001/jama.2020.14978.

Kaufman Hall. 2018. "2018 M&A in Review: A New Healthcare Landscape Takes Shape." mnareview.kaufmanhall.com/2018-m-a-in-review?_ga=2.181952807.180 3385474.1547482075-1258334907.1547482075 (accessed on May 3, 2021).

Khullar, Dhruv, Amelia M. Bond, and William L. Schpero. 2020. "COVID-19 and the Financial Health of US Hospitals." *JAMA* 323, no. 21: 2127–28. doi.org/10.1001/ jama.2020.6269.

Kinney, Eleanor D., and Bonnie Lefkowitz. 1982. "Capital Cost Reimbursement to Community Hospitals under Federal Health Insurance Programs." *Journal of Health Politics, Policy and Law* 7, no. 3: 648–66. doi.org/10.1215/03616878-7-3-648.

Liss, Samantha. 2020. "Nonprofit Health Systems—Despite Huge Cash Reserves—Get Billions in CARES Funding." Healthcare Dive, June 23. www.healthcaredive .com/news/nonprofit-health-systems-despite-huge-cash-reserves-get-billions-in -car/580078/.

Ly, Dan P., and David M. Cutler. 2018. "Factors of US Hospitals Associated with Improved Profit Margins: An Observational Study." *Journal of General Internal Medicine* 33, no. 7: 1020–27. doi.org/10.1007/s11606-018-4347-4.

MedPAC (Medicare Payment Advisory Commission). 2020. "Report to the Congress: Medicare Payment Policy." March. www.medpac.gov/docs/default-source/reports /mar20_entirereport_sec.pdf?sfvrsn=0.

NCRHRP (North Carolina Rural Health Research Program). 2020. "Most Rural Hospitals Have Little Cash Going into COVID." Findings Brief, May 11. www .shepscenter.unc.edu/?s=most+rural+hospitals+have+little+cash.

Pallone, Frank, Jr., and Richard E. Neal. 2020. Letter to HHS Secretary Alex M. Azar II and CMS Administrator Seema Verma. May 7. waysandmeans.house.gov/sites /democrats.waysandmeans.house.gov/files/documents/HHS.CMS_.%202020.5.7 .%20Letter%20re%20Provider%20Fund%20and%20Advance%20Payments.HE_ .pdf.

Pauly, Mark. 2019. "Will Health Care's Immediate Future Look a Lot Like the Recent Past? More Public-Sector Funding, but More Private-Sector Delivery and Admin-istration." American Enterprise Institute, June 7. www.aei.org/research-products /report/health-care-public-sector-funding/.

Pope, Chris. 2019. "The Cost of Hospital Protectionism." *National Affairs*, January 3. www.nationalaffairs.com/publications/detail/the-cost-of-hospital-protectionism.

Rau, Jordan. 2020. "Amid Coronavirus Distress, Wealthy Hospitals Hoard Millions." *Kaiser Health News*, April 28. khn.org/news/amid-coronavirus-distress-wealthy-hospitals-hoard-millions/.

Relman, Arnold S. 1980. "The New Medical-Industrial Complex." *New England Journal of Medicine* 303, no. 17: 963–70. doi.org/10.1056/nejm198010233031703.

Rosenthal, Elisabeth. 2019. "Analysis: How Your Beloved Hospital Helps to Drive Up Health Care Costs." *Kaiser Health News*, September 5. khn.org/news/analysis-how-your-beloved-hospital-helps-to-drive-up-health-care-costs/.

Schatzkin, Arthur. 1984. "The Relationship of Inpatient Racial Composition and Hospital Closure in New York City." *Medical Care* 22, no. 5: 379–87. doi.org/10.1097/00005650-198405000-00002.

Schwartz, Karen, and Anthony Damico. 2020. "Distribution of CARES Act Funding among Hospitals." Kaiser Family Foundation, May 13. www.kff.org/coronavirus-covid-19/issue-brief/distribution-of-cares-act-funding-among-hospitals/.

Serwer, Adam. 2009. "The De-Facto Segregation of Health Care." *American Prospect*, August 21. prospect.org/article/de-facto-segregation-health-care/.

Siegrist, Richard B., Jr. 1983. "Wall Street and the For-Profit Hospital Management Companies." In *The New Health Care for Profit: Doctors and Hospitals in a Competitive Environment*, edited by Bradford H. Gray, 35–50. Washington, DC: National Academy Press.

Soss, Joe, Richard C. Fording, and Sanford F. Schram. 2011. *Disciplining the Poor: Neoliberal Paternalism and the Persistent Power of Race*. Chicago: University of Chicago Press.

Stevens, Robert, and Rosemary Stevens. 1974. *Welfare Medicine in America: A Case Study of Medicaid*. New York: Free Press.

White, Chapin, Amelia M. Bond, and James D. Reschovsky. 2013. "High and Varying Pices for Privately Insured Patients Underscore Hospital Market Power." *Research Brief* 27: 1–10.

Yang, Tse-Chuan, Yunhan Zhao, and Qian Song. 2017. "Residential Segregation and Racial Disparities in Self-Rated Health: How Do Dimensions of Residential Segregation Matter?" *Social Science Research* 61: 29–42. doi.org/10.1016/j.ssresearch.2016.06.011.

State Policy and Mental Health Outcomes under COVID-19

Michael W. Sances
Temple University

Andrea Louise Campbell
Massachusetts Institute of Technology

Abstract

Context: The COVID-19 pandemic has caused enormous damage to physiological health and economic security, especially among racial and ethnic minorities. We examined downstream effects on mental health, how effects vary by race and ethnicity, and the role of existing state-level social policies in softening the pandemic's impact.

Methods: We analyze an online, multi-wave Census Bureau survey fielded to nearly a million respondents between late April and July 2020. The survey includes questions measuring psychological distress as well as indirect measures of experience with the pandemic. We combined these data with state-level measures of COVID-19 cases, lockdown orders, unemployment filings, and safety net policy.

Findings: We find significant mental stress among all respondents and a sizeable gap between nonwhite and white respondents. Adjusting for pandemic experiences eliminates this gap. The effect of losing work as a result of the pandemic is slightly offset by state policies such as unemployment benefit size and Medicaid expansion. The magnitude of these offsetting effects is similar across racial/ethnic groups.

Conclusions: The racialized impacts of the pandemic are exacerbated by inequalities in state policy exemplifying structural racism. If the least generous states matched the policies of the most generous, inequalities caused by the pandemic would be diminished.

Keywords COVID-19, mental health, race, structural racism

The COVID-19 pandemic has created both a public health crisis in the United States, with millions sickened and thousands dead, and an economic crisis, with unprecedented numbers of Americans facing furloughs or job loss and confronting food insecurity, housing insecurity, and the loss

Journal of Health Politics, Policy and Law, Vol. 46, No. 5, October 2021
DOI 10.1215/03616878-9155991 © 2021 by Duke University Press

of health insurance. At the same time, the pandemic response in the United States has been highly decentralized. Although federal relief bills temporarily augmented the social safety net, much of the response was relegated to states and localities, where both existing and pandemic-related policy choices varied widely. In addition, the twin health and economic crises affected ethnic and racial minorities the most, raising questions about the adequacy of state policy to offset the devastating effects of the pandemic.

In addition to the direct impacts on health and economic security, preliminary signs show that the pandemic has also had an impact on Americans' mental health (Carey 2020). Early examinations comparing survey responses from 2018 and 2020 find that depression symptoms and generalized distress increased (Ettman et al. 2020; McGinty et al. 2020). It is likely that racial and ethnic minorities are disproportionately affected by these mental health effects, and some news coverage of the pandemic has supported this assertion (Pan 2020). Nonetheless, there is still little systematic analysis of mental health outcomes during the pandemic, and even less on the question of disparate impacts by race and ethnicity.

Also unclear is the extent to which state policies are able to offset the negative mental health impacts of the pandemic. Previous studies show that safety net policies can alleviate mental health distress associated with unemployment and food insecurity (Oddo and Mabli 2015; Rodriguez, Frongillo, and Chandra 2001). Questions arise about the effectiveness of existing social policies, given the great magnitude and speed of the pandemic's economic effects, the impact of state variation in social policy generosity, and possible disparate effects across racial and ethnic subgroups.

We utilize data from a unique Census Bureau study to assess mental health effects on vulnerable groups. Fielded between late April and July 2020, this multi-wave study consists of about 1 million cases and includes questions on mental health (symptoms of depression and anxiety) and pandemic-related work loss. We use these data to explore the prevalence of psychological distress during the pandemic and how these mental stresses differ by race and ethnicity. We then link the individual-level experiences to state-level policies, such as the generosity of unemployment benefits, the presence of any paid sick leave policy, and whether a state expanded Medicaid under the Affordable Care Act. We test whether the negative effect of reduced income on mental health is offset by any of these policies and whether these offsetting effects vary, in turn, by race or ethnicity.

We find that the pandemic has had significant deleterious effects on Americans' mental health, with large majorities reporting symptoms of anxiety and depression. The negative mental health effects have been the most acute for Hispanic and Black Americans, with Asian and white

Americans faring relatively better. We also find that among all racial and ethnic groups, pandemic-related work loss worsens psychological distress and that existing state safety net policies ameliorate these effects only partially. We detect no substantive difference in these offsetting effects by race or ethnicity.

Studying whether existing state policies have helped offset the mental health effects of the pandemic is important, as it speaks to the potential need for future policy interventions. It also exposes the toll of state policy variation. Two otherwise similar individuals with the same loss of work income can experience different levels of psychological distress, depending merely on where they happen to live. This variation is deeply embedded in the racial politics of American social policy, which gave rise to interstate differences in safety net generosity and which continues to drive the disparate racial impacts of the pandemic.

Racial/Ethnic Minorities, Pandemic Experiences, and Mental Health

Pre-pandemic findings about the prevalence of psychological distress in the United States and the effects of economic downturns suggest the pandemic may have had substantial negative effects on individuals' well-being. Depression is the leading cause of disability in the United States to begin with (McKenna 2005), and economic recessions are associated with negative mental health outcomes both in the United States and abroad (Frasquilho et al. 2016; Mucci et al. 2016). With the pandemic leading to the highest levels of unemployment since the Great Depression and the most sudden increases in joblessness on record (Chaney and Morath 2020), journalistic accounts have warned of a looming mental health crisis (e.g., Wan 2020). Between the shutdowns, economic distress, and health worries, there are several reasons to suppose that symptoms of depression and anxiety rose during the pandemic.

A further possibility is that mental health outcomes during the pandemic were worse for vulnerable groups such as racial and ethnic minorities, given they experienced more severe physical health and economic effects on average than whites. Black and Hispanic Americans were more likely than whites to have the comorbidities that exacerbate COVID-19 (Golestaneh et al. 2020; Kabarriti 2020) and less likely to have health insurance (Artiga, Orgera, and Damico 2020). Black and Hispanic individuals were more likely to contract COVID-19 and to die from it, with particularly high mortality rates among African Americans (Webb Hooper, Napoles, and Perez-Stable 2020).

Racial and ethnic minority groups also confronted the worst of the pandemic's economic fallout. Black and Hispanic Americans experienced the highest unemployment rates, followed by Asian Americans, due in part to concentration in occupations and sectors most affected by economic shutdowns. In the second quarter of 2020, when unemployment peaked, the unemployment rate was 17.0% for Hispanics, 16.3% for African Americans, 14.4% for Asians, and 12.2% for whites, figures that were 9 to 13 percentage points higher than a year earlier (US Bureau of Labor Statistics 2020). Food insecurity also surged during the pandemic, with the proportion of households with children reporting food insecurity increasing most sharply for Black and Hispanic households, to 30% and 25%, respectively, in June 2020, compared to 15% for Asian households and less than 10% among white households (Bauer 2020).

Because poor physical health and economic stress are associated with negative mental health outcomes (Mucci et al. 2016; Ohrnberger, Fichera, and Sutton 2017), we might hypothesize that racial and ethnic minority groups who faced the brunt of the pandemic would report more psychological distress than white individuals. Clinical diagnosis of major depressive disorder is less common for Black Americans than among whites, raising concerns that symptomology and diagnosis rates may differ by race (Barnes and Bates 2017). However, Black and Hispanic individuals typically report similar or somewhat higher levels of generalized psychological distress than whites in survey-based instruments such as the Kessler 6 scale and the Patient Health Questionnaire (PHQ-2) and Generalized Anxiety Disorder (GAD-2) scales, which squares with the higher known prevalence of mental health stressors experienced by minority groups (Barnes and Bates 2017). In the National Health Interview Survey for 2015–16, for example, the percentage of adults with "serious psychological distress"—scoring 13 or higher on the 24-point Kessler 6 scale—was similar for non-Hispanic white (3.7%), Black (3.6%), and Hispanic (3.7%) individuals (NCHS 2018). A study conducted during the pandemic using the same measure found that severe psychological distress increased between 2018 and July 2020 for all racial/ethnic groups, with the largest increase among Hispanics (McGinty et al. 2020). Measuring psychological distress using modified versions of the PHQ-2 and GAD-2 scales, we report below large increases between April and July 2020 and much higher distress among Black and Hispanic individuals. One question is what pandemic-related stressors are driving these results. Another is how effective state safety net policies are in ameliorating their mental health effects.

Social Policies and Mental Health

Studies show food insecurity is associated with depression (Liu et al. 2014) but that participation in the Supplemental Nutrition Assistance Program (SNAP) reduces psychological distress in households followed over time (Oddo and Mabli 2015). Similarly, causal studies using panel data show increases in psychological distress and diagnosed mental disorders among unemployed workers (Farre, Fasani, and Mueller 2018), but unemployed women receiving unemployment benefits or other entitlement benefits have rates of depression similar to those of the employed (while unemployed men and women receiving means-tested benefits or no benefits reported higher rates of depression [Rodriguez, Frongillo, and Chandra 2001]). These studies suggest that government safety net programs can have a protective effect on the mental health of individuals facing economic insecurity. We explore whether such programs were able to provide such protective effects during the COVID-19 pandemic, given the speed and depth of the pandemic-induced economic decline. In addition, many safety net programs in the United States are run jointly by state and federal governments, with policy parameters that vary across the states, raising questions about cross-state differences in such protective effects. Unemployment insurance is a joint federal-state program, but eligibility, benefit levels, and duration vary across states. A few states have paid sick leave policies. Many states had expanded Medicaid under the Affordable Care Act, but 15 states did not have expansion in place in spring/summer 2020.[1]

Several mechanisms may link state social policies and individuals' mental health. Unemployment insurance helps offset income loss arising from job loss, reducing the financial strain that has been found to be a predictor of psychological distress among the unemployed (Kessler, Turner, and House 1987). Paid sick leave policies could similarly reduce financial strain by partly offsetting income loss among those who fell ill and could not work; studies show that individuals with access to paid sick leave report less psychological distress than those without (Stoddard-Dare et al. 2018). Medicaid expansion enhances the availability of health insurance for those whose employers do not offer insurance and for those who lost their jobs and therefore their insurance; those who are insured report less stress than the uninsured (APA 2017).

---

1. Thirty-eight states plus Washington, DC, had adopted Medicaid expansion as of October 1, 2020, but in three, adoption was effective after spring/summer 2020: Nebraska (planned for October 1, 2020), Oklahoma (planned for July 1, 2021), and Missouri (planned for July 1, 2021) (KFF 2020).

Although we do not have direct evidence on mechanisms, our data allow us to assess whether variations in the availability and generosity of these safety net programs across states are associated with lower levels of psychological distress among those experiencing job loss or diminished work during the coronavirus pandemic of 2020. Given that Black and Hispanic Americans have experienced the greatest economic fallout, we expect their mental health to be worse on average than white Americans'. We do not have a priori expectations about whether any offsetting effects of safety net policies differ in magnitude for minority groups compared to whites. But to the extent to which Black Americans in particular disproportionately live in states with the least expansive social policies—a reality resulting from the racist origins of state policy choices—they may benefit least from any offsetting effects.

Data and Measures

We use data from phase 1 of the Household Pulse Survey (HPS) conducted by the US Census Bureau, which consists of 12 weekly cross-sectional surveys from April 23 to July 21, 2020. Respondents are recruited by first sampling from the Census Bureau's master address file (MAF), then contacted by text and/or email and recruited into a Qualtrics survey. Responses were collected during a period when the economic fallout of the pandemic was most acute; the unemployment rate, which had been 3.5% in February 2020 and 4.4% in March, rose to 14.7% in April and remained elevated, at 13.3% in May, 11.1% in June, and 10.2% in July. The number of COVID-19 cases had a local peak around 30,000 per day in late April when the survey began, declined through the first week in June, then increased again to nearly 63,000 per day on the last day of data collection in late July (WHO 2020).

The Pulse Survey included four items assessing respondents' mental wellness, a modified version of the two-item PHQ-2 and the two-item GAD-2 scales measuring generalized psychological distress that appear in unmodified form on the National Health Interview Survey. Respondents were asked how often during the last seven days they had been bothered by "feeling nervous, anxious, or on edge"; "not being able to stop or control worrying"; "having little interest or pleasure in doing things"; and "feeling down, depressed, or hopeless." Each question has four response options: (1) not at all, (2) several days, (3) more than half the days, and (4) nearly every day. Although two of the items measure symptoms of anxiety and two depression, the four measures are highly correlated over time in our sample. At the individual level, the correlations between the four items range from 0.63 for the *interest* and *anxious* measures to 0.80 for the *anxious* and *worry* measures (anxiety and depression are often comorbid [Kessler et al. 2003]). In the findings below, we combine the four indicators into a single summary measure (online appendix A replicates tables 1–3 below for each of the four outcome variables separately; the results are largely the same as those for the combined measure).

We measure the state-level impact of the pandemic in three ways. First, we construct a measure of new COVID-19 cases by state using data from the *New York Times*. We compute daily new cases as the difference in new cases from day 1 to day 2; we then average the daily change in cases by week to merge it with the weekly survey data. We then log the new state cases measure. Second, we use the log number of total unemployment claims filed per week by state, from the US Department of Labor. Third, we use a time-varying measure of whether a state had an active shelter-in-place order when the respondent was surveyed; we obtain this measure from a database constructed by scholars at Boston University's School of Public Health (Raifman et al. 2020).

To capture the individual-level impacts of the pandemic, we use three measures. First, the HPS survey asks if anyone in the respondent's household experienced a loss of any employment income since March 13, 2020.[2] Second, while the survey does not ask if anyone in the household was sick with COVID-19, it does ask about not working in the past week because of being "sick with coronavirus symptoms." Third, we use a measure of the increase in food insecurity pre- and post-pandemic. The survey asks respondents which of the following characterizes their household's food situation prior to and subsequent to March 13: (1) enough of the kinds of food we wanted to eat; (2) enough, but not always the kinds of food we wanted to eat; (3) sometimes not enough to eat; (4) often not enough to eat. We compute the difference between the scales for post- and pre-March 13.

To study the impact of state policy, we use four measures of policy that we expect could offset the effect of pandemic-related work loss on

---

2. Note that this is a household-level measure and encompasses any reduction in income as a result of any lost work among any household member since March. The survey also includes a measure of whether a respondent themselves worked at all in the past week. We prefer the former measure, as we believe it does a better job of capturing the economic shock of the pandemic. For instance, many respondents might have seen reductions in work hours, but they would be coded as working in the past week by the latter measure. That said, our results are substantively similar when using the alternative measure.

mental health. First, we use the state's "replacement rate," or the percent of employment income covered by unemployment benefits in that state; we obtain this measure from the federal Department of Labor. Second, we also measure unemployment generosity using the maximum weekly benefit amount per state, from the World Population Review (state variation in state unemployment insurance [UI] benefits remains even after the $600 federal supplement contained in the CARES Act pandemic relief bill, signed March 27, 2020). Third, we use an indicator for whether a state has any paid sick leave policy, from the National Partnership for Women and Families. Fourth, we use an indicator for whether the state expanded its Medicaid program under the Affordable Care Act, from the Kaiser Family Foundation.[3]

While the Pulse data are valuable, given the timing and sample size, we note several limitations before proceeding. First, we are only able to classify respondents as Hispanic/White, Non-Hispanic/White, Black, Asian, or "Other." This means we cannot directly analyze responses among Native Americans, who may have been especially affected by the pandemic. Second, the mental health measures we employ are not directly comparable to the standard PHQ-2 and GAD-2 scales because they measure symptoms over the course of 7 days rather than the usual 14 days. Third, all our data are observational, and we are unable to leverage any temporal variation in social policy or individual-level experiences. Thus while the differences in the effects of lost wages may represent the causal effects of social policy, they may also represent other systematic differences between states.

Trends in Mental Health and Differences by Race/Ethnicity

Figure 1 plots the share of respondents reporting any adverse mental health (i.e., a 2, 3, or 4 on the original scale) for each of our four measures.[4] In

---

3. Nonwhite respondents may also have experienced increased mental distress as a result of the murder of George Floyd and a renewed focus on racism, after May 25 (e.g., Ang 2021; Bor et al. 2018). In online appendix C, we assess whether the murder of George Floyd and subsequent protests changed the trend in our mental health index and whether any break varied by racial group. We find mental distress worsened for Black respondents after May 25, but only by a small amount that is dwarfed by the overall racial gap.

4. Note that figure 1 shows any adverse mental health on any of the four indicators, not a score of 3 or more on the PHQ-2 (the cutpoint for screening for major depressive disorder) or 3 or more on the GAD-2 (the cutpoint for screening for generalized anxiety order) (CDC 2021).

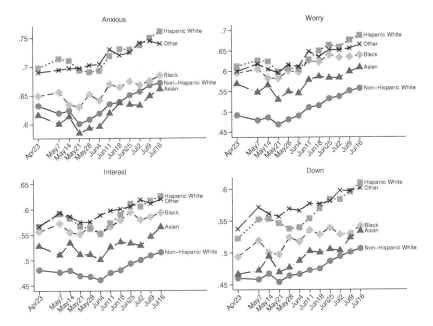

Figure 1 Psychological distress and race/ethnicity by week.

Note: The vertical axis is the share of respondents reporting any mental health stress on each of the four indicators.

each panel, we plot the share for each of five racial/ethnic groups, by survey week. Respondents reported extraordinarily high—and increasing—levels of psychological distress between April and July 2020. Even among the most sanguine respondents—non-Hispanic whites early in the survey period—over 45% reported symptoms of depression, and more than 60% reported feeling anxious. Ethnic and racial minority groups experienced even more mental health stress, with Hispanic respondents reporting the highest level of anxiety and depression followed by "Other" and Black respondents. White respondents reported the lowest levels, with Asians similar to whites or slightly elevated. Psychological distress increased significantly among all groups during this period, even though the unemployment rate and COVID-19 cases were falling.

We use a series of regressions to assess the statistical significance of these differences and to explore how much they are driven by the pandemic versus other factors. First, we combine all four measures of mental distress into a single measure, simply averaging the four four-point items. Second, we regress this measure on indicators for each racial/ethnic group, and indicators for survey week. Given possible serial correlation within states, and our interest in state-level policy factors, we cluster all standard errors at the state level.

The first column of table 1 mirrors the results in figure 1. Compared to the baseline of white respondents, Black respondents' self-reported mental distress is 0.127 (standard error of 0.011) higher on a four-point scale. Likewise, Hispanics' mental distress is 0.169 (0.006) higher, Asians' mental distress is 0.010 (0.011) higher (so not statistically significant), and mental distress among respondents classified as Other race/ethnicity is 0.216 (0.010) higher. To put these estimates in context, the standard deviation of our dependent variable is about 0.76.

In column 2, we begin to explore the drivers of these gaps, including state-level measures of new COVID-19 cases, unemployment filings, and shelter-in-place orders. Both COVID-19 cases and unemployment filings are significantly associated with greater psychological distress, while the estimate for lockdown orders is also positive but just shy of conventional levels of statistical significance. In column 3, we add individual-level experiences with the pandemic: losing work as a result of COVID-19 symptoms, losing any work income since March, and increased food insecurity. As predicted, all are significantly associated with worse mental health outcomes. For instance, losing any work income since March is associated with a 0.314 (standard error of 0.005) increase in mental distress. Notably, adjusting for these individual experiences lessens the racial gaps between whites and other groups; for example, the coefficient for Black is now 0.075.

In column 4, we add controls for having health insurance, having any school-age children, being married, income (an eight-point, ordinal scale we enter linearly), gender, and age in years. Interestingly, the inclusion of these variables almost entirely eliminates any mental health gaps between whites and Hispanics, and in two cases (for Blacks and Asians) the sign actually reverses. We interpret this result as evidence that variables such as income and having health insurance are, themselves, proxies for exposure to the pandemic. Once we adjust for these factors, we have essentially "controlled away" the pandemic's unequal impact, and so we have also controlled away the effect of race and ethnicity. This is not to say that race and ethnicity do not have an effect; rather, the deleterious mental health effects of the pandemic operate through nonwhites' greater economic insecurity. (Interestingly, but for reasons we cannot explore because of data limitations, the coefficient for the "Other" racial/ethnic category remains positive and significant, though reduced in magnitude.)

Table 1 Psychological Distress and Race/Ethnicity

	(1)	(2)	(3)	(4)
Black	0.127***	0.117***	0.075***	−0.064***
	(0.011)	(0.011)	(0.009)	(0.006)
Hispanic	0.169***	0.157***	0.107***	−0.000
	(0.006)	(0.005)	(0.008)	(0.011)
Asian	0.010	−0.001	−0.011	−0.033**
	(0.011)	(0.009)	(0.009)	(0.009)
Other	0.216***	0.217***	0.167***	0.067***
	(0.010)	(0.008)	(0.008)	(0.006)
Log new cases in state		0.009*	0.012**	0.008*
		(0.004)	(0.004)	(0.003)
Log state unemployment claims		0.011*	0.002	0.017**
		(0.005)	(0.005)	(0.006)
State shelter in place order		0.025	0.019	0.033**
		(0.013)	(0.012)	(0.010)
Lost work because had Covid			0.342***	0.242***
			(0.016)	(0.015)
Reduced household income			0.314***	0.238***
			(0.005)	(0.005)
Change in food insecurity			0.178***	0.157***
			(0.003)	(0.002)
Have health insurance				−0.072***
				(0.005)
Any school age kids				−0.012**
				(0.004)
Married				−0.080***
				(0.003)
Income				−0.054***
				(0.002)
Female				0.139***
				(0.002)
Age				−0.008***
				(0.000)
Constant	1.519***	1.328***	1.289***	1.881***
	(0.008)	(0.043)	(0.046)	(0.061)
Observations	987,139	987,139	980,303	930,284

Note: Regressions also include indicators for survey week; standard errors are in parentheses clustered by state.
 * p < .05, ** p < .01, *** p < .001.

Aside from associations with race and ethnicity, we find that lower-income, female, and younger respondents reported greater psychological distress compared to their higher-income, male, and older counterparts, in keeping with previous literature on the demographic correlates of mental health distress (Accortt, Freeman, and Allen 2008; Goldman, Glei, and Weinstein 2018; Weinberger et al. 2017). Being married and having children in the household have a protective effect, again in line with previous findings (Artazcoz et al. 2004; Jace and Makridis 2020).

The Role of State Policies

A key question is whether state social policies are able to offset the economic fallout—and in turn the negative mental health effects—of the pandemic. Table 2 evaluates the effect of four policies that vary across states: unemployment insurance replacement rates, maximum unemployment insurance benefits, the presence of paid sick leave, and Medicaid expansion under the Affordable Care Act (unsure which measure of unemployment benefit generosity would be most salient, we tested both). Because these policies do not vary over time, and because we are also interested in the effect of the policies on those directly impacted by the pandemic, we study policy effects using a series of regressions with interactions. That is, we regress our psychological distress index on an indicator for losing any income since March, the policy in question, and an interaction between losing income and the policy. The key quantity of interest is the interaction term, which tells us the difference between the effect of losing work income in states with one value of the policy and the effect of losing work income in states with another value of the policy. The "main" terms are less interesting but tell us the effect of losing work income in a state with the baseline level of the policy (the *reduced household income* coefficient) and the difference in average mental health outcomes between states with different values of the policy, among those not losing work (the *policy* coefficient).

Each regression in table 2 also includes all of the covariates from table 1, not shown for space reasons. The interaction term in the final row shows that, while the UI replacement rate has no effect (we suspect the proportion of employment income replaced is less salient to individuals than absolute benefit amount), the other three policies do offset the negative mental health effects of reduced income. Specifically, in states with the largest maximum UI benefits, the effect of losing work on psychological distress is 0.044 (standard error of 0.016) lower than in states with the

Table 2 Interactions between State Policies and Reduced Household Income

	(1) Replacement rate	(2) Max benefit	(3) Paid sick leave	(4) Medicaid expansion
Reduced household income	0.247***	0.257***	0.246***	0.258***
	(0.013)	(0.009)	(0.005)	(0.007)
Policy	−0.007	0.012	0.055***	0.034***
	(0.020)	(0.021)	(0.009)	(0.008)
Reduced income × policy	−0.015	−0.044**	−0.029**	−0.027**
	(0.019)	(0.016)	(0.011)	(0.008)
Observations	930,284	930,284	930,284	930,284

Note: All regressions include covariates from table 1; state-clustered errors are in parentheses.
* $p < .05$, ** $p < .01$, *** $p < .001$.

smallest benefits. Likewise, in states with paid sick leave, the effect of reduced income is 0.029 (0.011) lower than in states without paid sick leave.[5] In states that expanded Medicaid, the effect of work loss is 0.027 (0.008) lower than in states that did not expand. Generally speaking, more generous social policies have a small but statistically significant offsetting effect on the mental health fallout of work loss.

Finally, given that ethnic and racial minorities have suffered poorer mental health outcomes during the pandemic than whites, we explore whether these policies' protective effects differ for nonwhites compared to whites. In table 3 we simplify the racial/ethnic categories by using a nonwhite dummy variable. The ameliorating effects of policy for whites are again seen in the interaction between reduced income and policy. The triple interaction in the last row indicates whether the policy effects differ between white and nonwhite respondents. The coefficients in this row indicate that these policies have roughly equal effects across whites and nonwhites. For two of the policies, the UI replacement rate and paid sick leave, the estimates are not significantly different than zero. For the remaining policies, the max UI benefit and Medicaid expansion,

---

5. Recall that the "losing work/work loss/reduced income" measure indicates loss of employment income in the household, not necessarily unemployment, for which paid sick leave would not apply. In online appendix B we examine whether state paid sick leave counteracts the effect of "not working for pay" because of having COVID-19. The effect is not statistically significant, perhaps because those who did not work in the last week because they had COVID-19 include a mix of the unemployed and the still employed, with only the latter group having access to paid sick leave.

Table 3 Interactions between State Policies, Work Loss, and Race/Ethnicity

	(1) Replacement rate	(2) Max benefit	(3) Paid sick leave	(4) Medicaid expansion
Reduced household income	0.265***	0.273***	0.255***	0.274***
	(0.015)	(0.011)	(0.006)	(0.009)
Policy	−0.009	0.018	0.061***	0.036***
	(0.020)	(0.022)	(0.010)	(0.008)
Nonwhite	−0.016	0.009	0.014	0.008
	(0.014)	(0.011)	(0.007)	(0.008)
Reduced × nonwhite	−0.062***	−0.060***	−0.041***	−0.060***
	(0.013)	(0.010)	(0.007)	(0.009)
Reduced × policy	−0.027	−0.055**	−0.024	−0.034**
	(0.022)	(0.019)	(0.014)	(0.011)
Nonwhite × policy	0.036	−0.006	−0.033*	−0.002
	(0.023)	(0.019)	(0.013)	(0.012)
Reduced × policy × nonwhite	0.035	0.042*	0.005	0.024*
	(0.018)	(0.018)	(0.011)	(0.011)
Observations	930,284	930,284	930,284	930,284

Note: All regressions include covariates from previous tables; state-clustered errors are in parentheses.
* $p < .05$, ** $p < .01$, *** $p < .001$.

the estimates are positive and significantly different than zero, though not large enough for us to rule out any offsetting effects for nonwhites.[6]

Discussion

Although we find substantively similar offsetting policy effects across racial and ethnic groups, this does not necessarily imply that the policies we examine play no role in reducing the pandemic-induced gap in mental health outcomes across groups. For example, we estimate that the baseline effect of losing work income (in table 2) is about 0.26 (on a four-point scale) in states that did not expand Medicaid, and that this effect is reduced by 0.034 points in states that did expand Medicaid. Given nonwhites are disproportionately likely to have lost income because of the pandemic,

6. For instance, with white respondents, the coefficient for reduced income × Medicaid expansion is −0.034, with a standard error of 0.011, suggesting that the effect of reduced income on distress is 0.034 lower for whites living in expansion states. The triple interaction for reduced income × policy × nonwhite, in turn, is 0.024, with a standard error of 0.011. The offsetting effect for nonwhites is thus −0.034 + 0.024 = −0.010.

the benefits of Medicaid expansion would, in theory, flow disproportionately to this group. An increase in the number of states expanding Medicaid would, according to our estimates, help narrow the mental health gap by race and ethnicity.

At the same time, nonwhite Americans are also spatially concentrated in states with the least generous social policies. For instance, in 2015, the Kaiser Family Foundation estimated that 3.1 million Americans fell into the Affordable Care Act "coverage gap," meaning they would be eligible for Medicaid expansion if their state did expand but would remain uninsured if their state did not. The share of these Americans who are Black or Hispanic is 56% (Artiga, Damico, and Garfield 2015). Although more states expanded Medicaid after 2015, 7 of the 11 states with the highest share of Black population had not done so by spring/summer 2020. These findings correspond with academic research showing that in states with larger Black populations, state welfare benefits are lower (Howard 1999; Soss et al. 2001), as are unemployment benefits (Bruch, Gornick, and van der Naald 2020).

The less generous safety net policies of some states represent yet another example of the structural racism that pervades American public policy (King and Smith 2005; Michener 2019). The COVID-19 pandemic led to worker illness, reduced incomes, and loss of health insurance, among other threats to well-being. Social policy aimed at these needs can offset the psychological distress arising from these forms of health and economic insecurity. But states vary widely in their generosity, for reasons deeply embedded in the racialized development of the American welfare state (Lieberman 1998). The psychological toll of the pandemic laid bare the shortcomings of these varying state policy paths.

Conclusion

Majorities of Americans reported symptoms of depression and anxiety during the COVID-19 pandemic, but the reported symptoms were greater among minority groups than among whites. Although similar measures typically reveal levels of psychological distress among Black and Hispanic individuals that are the same or somewhat elevated compared to whites, during the pandemic such individuals reported dramatically higher rates of distress. The greater prevalence of depression and anxiety symptoms among Black and Hispanic populations is concerning for many reasons, including the fact that minority individuals are half as likely as non-Hispanic whites to receive mental health treatment (Gonzalez et al. 2010).

These analyses also indicate that social welfare policies can ameliorate the effects of severe economic insecurity. Those who lost employment income in states with paid sick leave provisions, Medicaid expansion in place, and more generous unemployment benefits experienced less psychological impact than those losing work income in states with lower benefits or no policy at all. Thus social policy generosity is associated with individual well-being. Because symptoms of anxiety and depression affect social, occupational, and educational performance as well as political participation (Ojeda 2015), our study suggests that government policy choices affect individuals' mental health and ability to successfully navigate their personal, professional, and political lives.

In the United States, however, many social policy parameters vary across states, owing significantly to the fraught racial politics of enactment, in which the white Southern lawmakers whose votes were needed for passage insisted on state control of program eligibility and generosity to limit access for Black Americans (Lieberman 1998). These dynamics were evident during the creation of both unemployment insurance in the 1930s and Medicaid in the 1960s. Other policies, such as nationwide paid sick leave, never passed, and were only created later in a handful of Democratic-led states. Such dynamics wove racism into the structure of American social policy. The ensuing toll harms members of minority groups every day but becomes particularly acute during economic emergencies such as the COVID-19 pandemic. The dramatically increased distress that the pandemic visited on many Americans was alleviated somewhat in states with more generous social policies. Unfortunately, Black Americans in particular are less likely to live in such states. If the least generous states matched the policies of the most generous, the negative mental health effects of the pandemic would be diminished.

■ ■ ■

Michael W. Sances is an assistant professor of political science at Temple University. He studies representation and accountability through the lens of US state and local governments. Recent research projects include the impact of the Affordable Care Act on political behavior, the causes and consequences of cities' use of fines and fees as a revenue source, and ideological voting in mayoral elections. He previously served as a postdoctoral scholar at Vanderbilt University and an assistant professor at the University of Memphis.
msances@temple.edu

Andrea Louise Campbell is the Sloan Professor of Political Science at MIT. Her interests include American politics, political behavior, public opinion, political inequality, and policy feedback. She is the author of *How Policies Make Citizens: Senior Citizen Activism and the American Welfare State* (2003); *The Delegated Welfare State: Medicare, Markets, and the Governance of Social Policy*, with Kimberly J. Morgan (2011); and *Trapped in America's Safety Net: One Family's Struggle* (2014). Funders include the National Science Foundation, the Robert Wood Johnson Foundation, and the Russell Sage Foundation. She is a member of the American Academy of Arts and Sciences.

Acknowledgments

We are grateful to the editors and two anonymous reviewers for their helpful feedback.

References

Accortt, Eynav Elgavish, Marlene P. Freeman, and John J. B. Allen. 2008. "Women and Major Depressive Disorder: Clinical Perspectives on Causal Pathways." *Journal of Women's Health* 17, no. 10: 1583–90.

Ang, Desmond. 2021. "The Effects of Police Violence on Inner-City Students." *Quarterly Journal of Economics* 136, no. 1: 115–68.

APA (American Psychological Association). 2017. "Stress in America: The State of Our Nation." November 1. www.apa.org/news/press/releases/stress/2017/state-nation.pdf.

Artazcoz, Lucía, Joan Banach, Carme Borrell, and Immaculada Cortès. 2004. "Unemployment and Mental Health: Understanding the Interactions among Gender, Family Roles, and Social Class." *American Journal of Public Health* 94, no. 1: 82–88.

Artiga, Samantha, Anthony Damico, and Rachel Garfield. 2015. "The Impact of the Coverage Gap for Adults in States Not Expanding Medicaid by Race and Ethnicity." Kaiser Family Foundation, October 26. www.kff.org/racial-equity-and -health-policy/issue-brief/the-impact-of-the-coverage-gap-in-states-not-expanding -medicaid-by-race-and-ethnicity/.

Artiga, Samantha, Kendal Orgera, and Anthony Damico. 2020. "Changes in Health Coverage by Race and Ethnicity since the ACA, 2010–2018." Kaiser Family Foundation, March 5. www.kff.org/racial-equity-and-health-policy/issue-brief/changes-in -health-coverage-by-race-and-ethnicity-since-the-aca-2010-2018/.

Barnes, David M., and Lisa M. Bates. 2017. "Do Racial Patterns in Psychological Distress Shed Light on the Black-White Depression Paradox? A Systematic Review." *Social Psychiatry and Psychiatric Epidemiology* 52, no. 8: 913–28.

Bauer, Lauren. 2020. "About 14 Million Children in the US Are Not Getting Enough to Eat." *Up Front* (blog), Brookings Institution, July 9. www.brookings.edu/blog/up -front/2020/07/09/about-14-million-children-in-the-us-are-not-getting-enough-to-eat.

Bor, Jacob, Atheendar S. Venkataramani, David R. Williams, and Alexander C. Tsai. 2018. "Police Killings and Their Spillover Effects on the Mental Health of Black Americans: A Population-Based, Quasi-Experimental Study." *Lancet* 392, no. 10144: 302–10.

Bruch, Sarah K., Janet C. Gornick, and Joseph van der Naald. 2020. "Geographic Inequality in Social Provision: Variation across the US States." Paper presented at the Conference on Research in Income Wealth, Hyatt Regency, Bethesda, MD, March 5–6. www.nber.org/system/files/chapters/c14438/c14438.pdf.

Carey, Benedict. 2020. "Is the Pandemic Sparking Suicide?" *New York Times*, May 19. www.nytimes.com/2020/05/19/health/pandemic-coronavirus-suicide-health.html.

CDC (Centers for Disease Control and Prevention). 2021. "Anxiety and Depression: Household Pulse Survey." National Center for Health Statistics, February 10. www .cdc.gov/nchs/covid19/pulse/mental-health.htm.

Chaney, Sarah, and Eric Morath. 2020. "April Unemployment Rate Rose to a Record 14.7%." *Wall Street Journal*, May 8. www.wsj.com/articles/april-jobs-report -coronavirus-2020-11588888089.

Ettman, Catherine K., Salma M. Abdalla, Gregory H. Cohen, Laura Sampson, Patrick M. Vivier, and Sandro Galea. 2020. "Prevalence of Depression Symptoms in US Adults before and during the COVID-19 Pandemic." *JAMA Network Open* 3, no. 9: e2019686. jamanetwork.com/journals/jamanetworkopen/fullarticle/2770146.

Farre, Lidia, Francesco Fasani, and Hannes Mueller. 2018. "Feeling Useless: The Effect of Unemployment on Mental Health in the Great Recession." *IZA Journal of Labor Economics* 7, no. 8: 1–34.

Frasquilho, Diana, Margarida Gaspar Matos, Ferdinand Salonna, Diogo Guerreiro, Claudia C. Storti, Tania Gaspar, and Jose M. Caldas-de-Almeida. 2016. "Mental Health Outcomes in Times of Economic Recession: A Systematic Literature Review." *BMC Public Health* 16, article no. 115. doi.org/10.1186/s12889-016-2720-y.

Goldman, Noreen, Dana A. Glei, and Maxine Weinstein. 2018. "Declining Mental Health among Disadvantaged Americans." *PNAS* 115, no. 28: 7290–95.

Golestaneh, Ladan, Joel Neugarten, Molly Fisher, Henny H. Billett, Morayma Reyes Gil, Tanya Johns, Milagros Yunes, et al. 2020. "The Association of Race and COVID-19 Mortality." *EClinicalMedicine* 25, no. 100455. www.thelancet.com/action/show Pdf?pii=S2589-5370%2820%2930199-1.

Gonzalez, Hector M., William A. Vega, David R. Williams, Wassim Tarraf, Brady T. West, and Harold W. Neighbors. 2010. "Depression Care in the United States: Too Little for Too Few." *Archives of General Psychiatry* 67, no. 1: 37–46.

Howard, Christopher. 1999. "The American Welfare State, or States?" *Political Research Quarterly* 52, no. 2: 421–42.

Jace, Clara, and Christos A. Makridis. 2020. "Will You Be Mine? Marriage as a Protective Factor during Coronavirus." SSRN, July 27. doi.org/10.2139/ssrn.3655856.

Kabarriti, Rafi, N. Patrik Brodin, Maxim I. Maron, Chandan Guha, Shalom Kalnicki, Madhur K. Garg, and Andrew D. Racine. 2020. "Association of Race and Ethnicity with Comorbidities and Survival among Patients with COVID-19 at an Urban Medical Center in New York." *JAMA Network Open* 3, no. 9: e2019795. jamanetwork.com /journals/jamanetworkopen/fullarticle/2770960.

Kessler, Ronald C., Patricia Berglund, Olga Demler, Robert Jin, Doreen Koretz, Kathleen R. Merikangas, A. John Rush, Ellen E. Walters, and Philip S. Wang. 2003. "The Epidemiology of Major Depressive Disorder: Results from the National Comorbidity Survey Replication (NCS-R)." *JAMA* 289, no. 23: 3095–3105.

Kessler, Ronald C., J. Blake Turner, and James S. House. 1987. "Intervening Processes in the Relationship between Unemployment and Health." *Psychological Medicine* 17, no. 4: 949–61.

KFF (Kaiser Family Foundation). 2020. "Status of State Action on the Medicaid Expansion Decision." October 1. www.kff.org/health-reform/state-indicator/state -activity-around-expanding-medicaid-under-the-affordable-care-act/?currentTime frame=0&sortModel=%7B%22colId%22:%22Location%22,%22sort%22:%22asc %22%7D.

King, Desmond S., and Rogers M. Smith. 2005. "Racial Orders in American Political Development." *American Political Science Review* 99, no. 1: 75–92.

Lieberman, Robert C. 1998. *Shifting the Color Line: Race and the American Welfare State*. Cambridge, MA: Harvard University Press.

Liu, Yong, Rashid S. Njai, Kurt J. Greenlund, Daniel P. Chapman, and Janet B. Croft. 2014. "Relationships between Housing and Food Insecurity, Frequent Mental Distress, and Insufficient Sleep among Adults in Twelve US States, 2009." *Preventing Chronic Disease*, March 13. doi.org/10.5888/pcd11.130334.

McGinty, Emma E., Rachel Presskreischer, Hahrie Han, and Colleen L. Barry. 2020. "Psychological Distress and Loneliness Reported by US Adults in 2018 and April 2020." *JAMA* 324, no. 1: 93–94.

McKenna, Matthew T. 2005. "Assessing the Burden of Disease in the United States using Disability-Adjusted Life Years." *American Journal of Preventive Medicine* 28, no. 5: 415–23.

Michener, Jamila. 2019. "Policy Feedback in a Racialized Polity." *Policy Studies Journal* 47, no. 2: 423–50.

Mucci, Nicola, Gabriele Giorgi, Mattia Roncaioli, Javier Fiz Perez, and Giulio Arcangeli. 2016. "The Correlation between Stress and Economic Crisis: A Systematic Review." *Neuropsychiatric Disease and Treatment* 12: 983–93.

NCHS (National Center for Health Statistics). 2018. *Health, United States, 2017: With Special Feature on Mortality*. Hyattsville, MD: NCHS.

Oddo, Vanessa M., and James Mabli. 2015. "Association of Participation in the Supplemental Nutrition Assistance Program and Psychological Distress." *American Journal of Public Health* 105, no. 6: 30–35.

Ohrnberger, Julius, Eleonora Fichera, and Matt Sutton. 2017. "The Relationship between Physical and Mental Health: A Mediation Analysis." *Social Science and Medicine* 195: 42–49.

Ojeda, Christopher. 2015. "Depression and Political Participation." *Social Science Quarterly* 96, no. 5: 1226–43.

Pan, Deanna. 2020. "Black Americans, Suffering Disproportionately from COVID-19, Face a Mounting Mental Health Crisis." *Boston Globe*, September 7. www .bostonglobe.com/2020/09/07/metro/black-americans-suffering-disproportionately -covid-19-face-mounting-mental-health-crisis/.

Raifman, Julia, Kristen Nocka, David Jones, Jacob Bor, Sarah Ketchen Lipson, Jonathan Jay, and Philip Chan. 2020. "COVID-19 US State Policy Database." www.tinyurl.com/statepolicies (accessed January 18, 2021).

Rodriguez, Eunice, Edward A. Frongillo, and Pinky Chandra. 2001. "Do Social Programmes Contribute to Mental Well-Being? The Long-Term Impact of Unemployment on Depression in the United States." *International Journal of Epidemiology* 30, no. 1: 163–70.

Soss, Joe, Sanford F. Schram, Thomas Vartanian, and Erin S. O'Brien. 2001. "Setting the Terms of Relief: Explaining State Policy Choices in the Devolution Revolution." *American Journal of Political Science* 45, no. 2: 378–95.

Stoddard-Dare, Patricia, Leaanne DeRigne, Cyleste C. Collins, Linda M. Quinn, and Kimberly Fuller. 2018. "Paid Sick Leave and Psychological Distress: An Analysis of US Workers." *American Journal of Orthopsychiatry* 88, no. 1: 1–9.

US Bureau of Labor Statistics. 2020. "Employment Status of the Civilian Noninstitutional Population by Race, Hispanic or Latino Ethnicity, Sex and Age, Seasonally Adjusted." www.bls.gov/web/empsit/cpsee_e02.pdf (accessed October 14, 2020).

Wan, William. 2020. "The Coronavirus Pandemic Is Pushing America into a Mental Health Crisis." *Washington Post*, May 4. www.washingtonpost.com/health/2020/05/04/mental-health-coronavirus/.

Webb Hooper, Monica, AnnaMaria Napoles, and Eliseo J. Perez-Stable. 2020. "COVID-19 and Racial/Ethnic Disparities." *JAMA* 323, no. 24: 2466–67.

Weinberger, Andrea H., Misato Gbedemah, A. M. Martinez, Denis Nash, Sandro Galea, and R. D. Goodwin. 2017. "Trends in Depression Prevalence in the USA from 2005 to 2015: Widening Disparities in Vulnerable Groups." *Psychological Medicine* 48, no. 8: 1308–15.

WHO (World Health Organization). 2020. "WHO Coronavirus Disease (COVID-19) Dashboard." covid19.who.int (accessed October 14, 2020).

The Treatment of Disability under Crisis Standards of Care: An Empirical and Normative Analysis of Change over Time during COVID-19

Ari Ne'eman
Michael Ashley Stein
Harvard University

Zackary D. Berger
Johns Hopkins University

Doron Dorfman
Syracuse University

Abstract

Context: COVID-19 has prompted debates between bioethicists and disability activists about Crisis Standards of Care plans (CSCs), triage protocols determining the allocation of scarce life-saving care.

Methods: We examine CSCs in 35 states and code how they approach disability, comparing states that have revised their plans over time to those that have not. We offer ethical and legal analyses evaluating to what extent changes to state policy aligned with disability rights law and ethics during the early pandemic and subsequently as stakeholder engagement grew.

Findings: While disability rights views were not well represented in CSCs that were not updated or updated early in the pandemic, states that revised their plans later in the pandemic were more aligned with advocate priorities. However, many CSCs continue to include concerning provisions, especially the reliance on long-term survival, which implicates considerations of both disability rights and racial justice.

Conclusions: The disability rights movement's successes in influencing state triage policy should inform future CSCs and set the stage for further work on how stakeholders influence bioethics policy debates. We offer thoughts for examining bioethics policy making reflecting the processes by which activists seek policy change and the tension policy makers face between expert delegation and mediating values conflicts.

Keywords COVID-19, bioethics, Crisis Standards of Care, disability rights, health law

As COVID-19 forces providers to decide how to triage scarce resources, disability activists and bioethicists have engaged in a robust debate on how to allocate treatment should demand exceed availability.

Journal of Health Politics, Policy and Law, Vol. 46, No. 5, October 2021
DOI 10.1215/03616878-9156005 © 2021 by Duke University Press

At the beginning of the pandemic, prominent bioethicists made the case for rationing care on the basis of disability, prompting criticism regarding the potential for discrimination and bias (Brown and Goodwin 2020; Emanuel et al. 2020). These rationing proposals built on a research literature developed during the last two decades regarding Crisis Standards of Care (CSC)—defined by the Institute of Medicine (IOM 2009) as "substantial change in the usual health care operations and the level of care it is possible to deliver, which is made necessary by a pervasive or catastrophic disaster." CSC plans (CSCs) articulate how to allocate scarce resources in the context of scarcity, giving providers instructions as to both the conservation of scarce resources and who shall receive them when there is not enough to go around. Many states had already adopted CSCs prior to the pandemic and others rapidly joined them as it became clear that COVID-19 would bring shortages of ventilators and other key medical resources.

While public health experts have long warned of the risk of widespread shortages of ventilators and other scarce resources in a public health emergency, prior to the emergence of COVID-19 state CSCs did not receive the same level of attention from civil rights advocates as other more imminent concerns. Consequently, policies developed prior to the pandemic were crafted primarily by bioethicists and clinicians with relatively little public scrutiny or engagement from stakeholder groups representing marginalized communities. These plans came under increased scrutiny only after COVID-19 prompted widespread shortages.

Disability groups have been on the forefront of such efforts because of the central role disability plays in CSC allocation criteria. Racial justice and aging groups have also engaged, often in collaboration with disability organizations (Network for Public Health Law 2020; Pressley 2020). Activists critiqued early calls from bioethicists to send disabled people to the "back of the line" through both explicit deprioritization and the application of ostensibly neutral criteria that disproportionately screened out disabled patients (Ne'eman 2020; Whyte 2020). These critiques reflect larger tensions between civil rights and clinical/bioethics frames for policy making regarding scarce resource allocation.

Such debates should both inform policy makers and contribute to a more robust understanding of how activists influence bioethics debates. This article advances ethical and legal arguments regarding how CSCs should approach disability, then provides an empirical analysis of how state CSC policies have evolved over the course of the pandemic. We also offer some initial thoughts to precipitate debate regarding processes of change in bioethics policy and the tension between expert delegation and stakeholder engagement in bioethics policy making.

How Does the Disability Rights Movement Approach Crisis Standards of Care Plans?

We begin by articulating the disability rights critique on CSC policy, informed both by our own analysis and the communications produced by activists over the course of the pandemic (CPR 2021; CPR and Bagenstos 2020). We articulate both ethical and legal issues for consideration in evaluating state CSCs. Two key principles guide our analysis: first, that when Congress passed Section 504 of the Rehabilitation Act and the Americans with Disabilities Act (ADA), it articulated a broad set of circumstances in which expending additional resources on people with disabilities, even when inefficient, is legally required (Ne'eman 2020; Pendo 2020); and second, that the purpose of emergency life-sustaining medical care is to save lives during acute care episodes, not to maximize life-years or make broader societal judgments regarding who is worthy of care.

Our analysis in the first part of this article is split into seven sections, informed by the empirical work reported in the second part. That work makes use of a dataset we developed of 58 state CSC policies from 35 states. State CSCs were reviewed to identify key points of policy variation relevant to people with disabilities. We found five domains in which we observed significant variation with respect to disability: (1) use of categorical exclusions, (2) use of long-term survival, (3) use of resource intensity, (4) protections against reallocation of personal ventilators, and (5) modifications to prognostic scoring instruments. In this section, we discuss two domains held in common across CSCs as well as the five domains in which we documented variation.

Quality of Life Judgments

One of the disability rights movement's earliest priorities during the pandemic was the rejection of quality of life judgments as an allocation criteria within CSC plans. In this, the movement has been successful—CSCs have avoided or prohibited quality of life judgments. This is a very straightforward application of disability rights law. Nonetheless, prohibiting quality of life judgments in CSCs represents an important victory, as they remain common in other areas of medical decision making, such as qualitative futility determinations and quality adjusted life year (QALY) calculations (NCD 2019). Though clinicians frequently rate disabled patients' quality of life as worse than that of nondisabled patients, this often conflicts with the perspectives of people with disabilities themselves

(Iezzoni et al. 2021; Stramondo 2021). Some CSCs have explicitly pro-hibited the use of the QALY and similar tools (Bateman et al. 2020). The clear rejection of quality of life as an appropriate CSC triage factor also helps open the door to long-overdue conversations on their appropriateness in non-pandemic decision making.

Short-Term Survival

Most CSCs make use of some assessment of short-term mortality risk to allocate resources. While standards of quantitative futility have long per-mitted clinicians to deny care deemed exceedingly unlikely to be effective, CSCs also allow prioritization by relative short-term mortality risk. Major disability groups agree that using relative short-term mortality risk is not illegal within a CSC context (CPR and Bagenstos 2020). We also agree, since survival to discharge from an acute care episode is part of the purpose of lifesaving medical care. Thus, while optimizing for life-years represents an unacceptable departure from the purpose of emergency care, optimizing for lives saved is consistent with it. However, we contend that short-term mortality risk should be interpreted narrowly to avoid unnecessarily screening out of individuals with disabilities and to reduce the risk of bias from more subjective longer-term judgments. Our preferred stan-dard would be survival to hospital discharge. Alternatively, a December 2020 joint statement from the National Academy of Medicine (NAM), the American Medical Association (AMA), and other major national medical associations has endorsed a similarly narrow standard, arguing that resource allocation decisions should be made based only on "like-lihood of death prior to or imminently after hospital discharge" (NAM 2020). This joint statement (hereafter referred to as the NAM statement) was an effort by major medical groups to communicate lessons learned on CSC policy over the course of the pandemic to the field, including information on compliance with civil rights law and best practices for avoiding bias and discrimination. It represented an important acknowl-edgment and validation of disability rights claims with respect to CSC policy making.

Categorical Exclusions

Exclusion criteria render whole categories of individuals with disabilities outside the scope of critical care, typically through restrictions on the basis of diagnosis and functional impairment. We argue that they are ethically wrong and legally impermissible. Many pre-pandemic CSCs incorporated categorical exclusions on the basis of particular diagnoses, sometimes in association with specific levels of functional impairment. Under such exclusions, individuals with these conditions are automatically excluded from accessing critical care resources.

Some CSC plans have justified exclusions by presuming that patients with specific conditions meet criteria that render them ineligible. For example, many CSCs with exclusion criteria appear to have copied them from the 2004 Ontario Health Plan for an Influenza Pandemic (OHPIP) (Christian et al. 2006). The OHPIP articulates three rationales for exclusion criteria: (1) low likelihood of short-term survival, (2) an anticipated high use of resources, and (3) a low likelihood of long-term survival. We contend that the use of categorical exclusions is inappropriate regardless of rationale (and, as articulated below, we argue that the latter two of these rationales are ethically and legally impermissible).

Disability rights law requires an individualized assessment prior to deeming a person unqualified for a program or service on the basis of disability, in part because evaluating whether someone is qualified must be done while accounting for reasonable modifications. This is as true for medical services as it is for any other service that people with disabilities wish to use.[1]

Some might argue that categorical exclusions may be appropriate in circumstances in which treatment is exceedingly unlikely to be effective for every individual in a given category. While such circumstances do occur, treatment that is exceedingly unlikely to be effective can be denied under existing standards of quantitative futility. Since CSCs exist to articulate circumstances in which care that would typically be provided would not be, categorical exclusions should not be made use of in a CSC context. Avoiding the use of categorical exclusion criteria is also entirely consistent with CSC conditions. The recent NAM (2020) statement instructs providers to "make resource allocation decisions based on individualized assessments of each patient ... such assessments should NOT use categorical exclusion criteria on the basis of disability or age."

Ironically, those opposing claims for systemic reasonable modifications for groups of people with disabilities often rely on the idea of individualized assessment, arguing that because each diagnosis comprises people with different needs, group-based claims for modifications are

---

1. *Bragdon v. Abbott*, 524 U.S. 624 (1998); *Sch. Bd. of Nassau Cty., Fla. v. Arline*, 480 U.S. 273 (1987); *United States v. Asare*, 2018 WL 2465378 (S.D.N.Y. 2018).

inappropriate and must be sought on an individualized basis rather than emerging solely from the fact of a diagnosis (Stein and Waterstone 2006). It would be perverse to insist that individualized assessment is required for a modification to assist people with disabilities while allowing disability-related penalties to be imposed based on group-based judgments without individualization.

Long-Term Survival

Many CSCs utilize prospects of long-term survival as a qualification for receipt of lifesaving medical treatment. In doing so, plans argue that this maximizes the number of "life-years" saved, whereas allocating on the basis of short-term mortality merely maximizes the number of lives saved.

In response, multiple ethical arguments have been advanced against the use of long-term survival as an allocation criterion. Others have pointed out that some life-limiting conditions are often the result of structural inequality, especially regarding race and class (Schmidt, Roberts, and Eneanya 2021). We concur and believe that disability should figure into that analysis as well, given that people with disabilities experience significant health disparities and bias from medical professionals (Iezzoni 2021; Krahn, Walker, and Correa-De-Araujo 2015). Although this does not address the permissibility of deprioritizing patients on the basis of life-limiting conditions that are not the result of structural inequality, we advance additional arguments for avoiding the use of long-term survival altogether.

First, within the same diagnosis, it is infeasible for physicians to determine whether a patient acquired the condition because of "structural" reasons as opposed to poor choices or random chance. Accepting such inquiries would also permit the allocation of medical care based on other judgments of personal behavior and moral worth (like denying care to patients whose conditions are the result of past smoking, obesity, or risk-taking behavior). Such an approach would corrode the equitable practice of medicine.

Some propose to avoid this assessment through the use of equity weights, prioritizing care to those from disadvantaged backgrounds by assigning numeric weights to forms of disadvantage (Schmidt, Roberts, and Eneanya 2021). Setting aside the legality of such an approach, doing so would necessitate quantifying the unquantifiable: policy makers would need to determine, with mathematical precision, the relative weight of each form of marginalized identity. A further alternative approach, assessing social disadvantage based on zip code, is worthwhile but insufficient in that it ignores forms of disadvantage that are not geographically congregated.

Second, even when dealing with diagnoses that were not acquired because of structural inequality, likelihood of survival is influenced by societal priorities. For example, life expectancy for people with cystic fibrosis and HIV/AIDS has increased dramatically as a result of research investments emerging from activism. Such instances demonstrate that the survival expectancy is not the result of random chance but is instead the result of societal choices about which conditions deserve investment.

Third, it is important to acknowledge that judgments of long-term survival are inherently uncertain and may be made using outdated information. This uncertainty is present even with condition-specific expert judgment and is compounded when such expertise is not available. Under such circumstances, clinicians may make decisions based on outdated information.

For example, many early CSCs included an exclusion criterion for cystic fibrosis with post-bronchodilator FEV1 < 30%, taken from the 2004 OHPIP exclusion criteria for conditions with "a baseline death rate higher than 50% within the next 1 to 2 years" (Christian et al. 2006). Tracing the citations that OHPIP relied on to ascertain that this exclusion met their stated rationale, we discovered its origins lie in a study by Eiten Kerem and colleagues (1992), which relied on cohort data from 1977 and 1989 (ASTP 1998). Unsurprisingly, life expectancy for people with cystic fibrosis has improved during the last 40 years. Even when the OHPIP criteria were developed, people with cystic fibrosis and post-bronchodilator FEV1 < 30% had a life expectancy above OHPIP's stated rationale (Milla and Warwick 1998).

This has far-reaching implications. That outdated life-expectancy judgments were propagated in many CSCs without further scrutiny calls into question whether such judgments will be made based on the best available objective medical evidence. Even where particular diagnoses are not singled out, many clinicians lack the expertise to assess prognosis for patients with uncommon disabilities on a truly individualized basis. This concern has been acknowledged in several CSCs that require at least two providers to assess individuals with certain diagnoses prior to a denial of care, preferably including one with condition-specific expertise (Bateman et al. 2020). Such a safeguard is advisable for mitigating risk of bias in short-term mortality assessments but is insufficient to justify use of long-term survival.

Finally, we argue that permitting the use of long-term life expectancy may violate federal disability rights laws. In evaluating the permissibility of denying modifications to requirements that disadvantage people with disabilities, disability laws inquire first whether the modification is necessary and reasonable as opposed to nonessential or significantly changing the nature of the program or service in question. If the requested modification would constitute a "fundamental alteration," it need not be provided. The ADA's prohibition of public entities using "eligibility criteria that screen out or tend to screen out an individual with a disability or any class of individuals with disabilities" is balanced against a showing that "such criteria can be shown to be necessary for the provision of the service, program, or activity being offered."[2]

In the context of life-sustaining treatment, the essential purpose of care is to maximize lives saved, not to maximize life-years. This holds true even under CSC conditions, as the NAM (2020) statement affirms in indicating that providers should not make use of "judgments as to long-term life expectancy." Accordingly, clinical determinations at the time of treatment should be based on saving or sustaining the lives of recipients, whether with or without preexisting disabilities, and should not be predicated on the unrelated issue of how long such individuals might survive after the provision of health care. To prevent discrimination under federal laws, medical providers must remain faithful to the purpose of life-sustaining care: simply to save lives.

Resource Intensity

While not as common as long-term survival, some CSCs allocate by resource intensity (sometimes referred to as duration of need). Those who argue for using resource intensity contend that failing to do so will result in fewer lives saved than using a strictly efficient allocation of care that deprioritizes those who require greater resources. This is true, but it fails to account for distributional implications.

As Joseph A. Stramondo (2020) points out, prohibiting the use of resource intensity "may be inefficient, but is surely not wasteful." Accepting some degree of inefficiency is embedded in disability rights law, which can require expending additional resources on reasonable accommodations and modifications in the name of equality of opportunity. We believe that the global adoption of this broad conception of nondiscrimination reflects an ethical norm in favor of accepting certain inefficiencies in the name of disability equality, not just a legal one.

It should also be noted that this is not a "blank check"; many people with disabilities will require modifications rising to a level of an undue burden or fundamental alteration of the program in question and thus be unqualified

---

2. 28 CFR § 35.130.

for those accommodations (Ne'eman 2020). But law and ethics both require some degree of modification, precluding a strict optimization approach that seeks only maximal efficiency.

This is true despite cases rejecting variation based on disability in certain contexts. The most prominent of these cases, *Alexander v. Choate*,[3] was handed down by the Supreme Court in 1985. The State of Tennessee reduced the annual number of paid hospital days for Medicaid patients from 20 to 14, without exception. The action was alleged to violate Section 504 because it would have a disproportionate impact on persons with disabilities who required a greater number of annual hospital days. The court rejected this challenge, ruling that as long as those with disabilities were not prevented "meaningful access" to the benefit, being affected differently by the same benefit did not constitute prohibited discrimination. This reasoning has been termed the access/content distinction (Bagenstos 2009).

The access/content distinction has been challenged on a number of grounds, most persuasively by Leslie Francis and Anita Silvers (2017). They argue that, according to *Choate*, the access/content distinction is constrained when the criteria for meaningful access is itself discriminatory for persons with disabilities. Hence, if doctors will not operate on an individual because she requires more than 14 days of hospital recovery, that action violates the patient's meaningful access. For patients with disabilities seeking treatment under conditions governed by a CSC, meaningful access is barred when care is predicated on discriminatory criteria. Thus disability rights laws are violated in instances in which clinicians will not provide the same care because a disabled patient will require greater post-care resources. In such cases, federal laws would compel the provision of reasonable modifications (including utilization of some additional resources) as part of those patients' equal access to health care.

It is unlikely that clinicians can evaluate future resource needs with enough precision to judge whether a particular patient's more intensive anticipated resource utilization is likely to be reasonable or whether a future patient is likely to have sufficiently less intense needs to justify reallocation. Evaluating if a reasonable modification might constitute a fundamental alteration or undue burden cannot be done without considering the resources available to the entity engaged in resource allocation (Stein 2003).[4] Notably, in the ever-shifting chaos of a pandemic, hospitals are not able to predict what the state of available resources will be days or

---

3. 469 U.S. 287 (1985).
4. 28 CFR 35.164; 28 CFR 36.104.

weeks in the future. As a result, CSCs should not prioritize by resource intensity. The NAM (2020) statement concurs, indicating that providers "should NOT deprioritize persons on the basis of disability or age because they may consume more treatment resources or require auxiliary aids or supports."

Criticizing disability activists, Govind Persad (2020) argues against concerns about relative allocation criteria, as policies deprioritizing patients with unfavored disabilities "would be expected to save more people with disabilities" overall. Responding to the argument that advocates should not abandon those subject to disability discrimination because other disabled people may benefit from discriminatory policies, David Wasserman, Persad, and Joseph Millum (2020) claim that such an approach constitutes "requiring solidarity with a specific group." We emphatically disagree.

Persad's approach would twist civil rights law beyond recognition, suggesting that individual members of protected classes cannot be discriminated against by a policy so long as more numerous members of the same class benefit in the aggregate (Bagenstos 2020). While protecting against group-based discrimination, civil rights laws create individual protections that all members of the group benefit from, even when they are not personally subject to discrimination. And where laws provide protection against discrimination that impacts only a minority of people with disabilities, advocates have every reason to maintain the right of each individual to make sound claims. Persad's purely aggregate approach to assessing nondiscrimination would relegate civil rights law to a transactional enterprise between groups, rather than a system of rights protecting individuals.

Reasonable Modifications

Most CSCs made use of the Sequential Organ Failure Assessment (SOFA) as their primary clinical instrument to assess short-term mortality risk for adults. The SOFA is a composite of different instruments, each of which contributes "points" to a patient's overall SOFA score, with higher scores indicative of greater risk of short-term mortality risk—and thus a lower relative priority for care. Such prognostic scoring systems have not been found to be reliable in the context of COVID-19 but nonetheless remain in common usage (NAM 2020).

In response to critiques from disability groups, a growing number of state CSC plans have articulated reasonable modifications to clinical instruments used to assess short-term mortality risk, most notably the SOFA. Disability rights law requires covered entities, including health care providers, to modify policies, practices, and procedures when necessary to afford access to individuals with disabilities, unless doing so would constitute a fundamental alteration of the service, program, or activity.

Modifications may be necessary when applying the SOFA and similar instruments designed to assess short-term mortality risk in acute conditions (Ne'eman 2020). Characteristics associated with stable underlying disabilities that are not predictive of short-term mortality may nonetheless result in an elevated score and thus inaccurately imply a greater risk of short-term mortality. The most frequently cited example of this concern is the Glasgow Coma Scale (GCS), one of several component instruments of the SOFA, which intends to measure acute brain injury severity. The GCS results in a more severe score for patients without intelligible speech or with impaired motor movement, giving such patients lower relative priority for resources. For patients with cerebral palsy, intellectual disability, or other underlying disabilities that interfere with speech and motor movement without greater mortality risk, unmodified use of the GCS deprioritizes inappropriately. Advocates have argued that CSCs should instruct providers to make modifications to clinical instruments to account for the needs of these patients. It would be difficult to argue that such modifications constitute a fundamental alteration when they ensure that clinical instruments are valid for the purpose they are designed to serve—assessing short-term mortality risk. Furthermore, the NAM (2020) statement notes the need to modify prognostic scoring systems "when necessary for accurate use with patients with underlying disabilities."

Some plans have articulated modifications beyond prognostic scoring systems. For example, Rhode Island's November 2020 update to its CSC discusses modifications in the context of therapeutic trials designed to assess ventilator effectiveness, noting that trial duration may need to be longer "for individuals with disabilities who may need additional time to demonstrate effective progress" (RIDOH 2020). We endorse this approach.

The concept of modifying the SOFA to address systemic inequalities has recently been expanded to encompass racial injustice. Harald Schmidt, Dorothy E. Roberts, and Nwamaka D. Eneanya (2021) note that the SOFA also disadvantages Black patients, in part because "creatinine is higher in Black communities because of higher rates of chronic kidney disease . . . the consequences of health inequities and structural racism." Massachusetts's most recent CSC revision sought to address this problem by indicating that patients with chronic kidney disease could be assigned only up to two points (instead of four) for elevated creatinine (Bateman et al. 2020). This represents a precedent-setting extension of the disability rights framework of reasonable modifications to other systemic inequities.

Chronic Ventilator Reallocation

Early in the pandemic, chronic ventilator users were concerned that CSCs permitting the reallocation of ventilators might result in the loss of technology they consider part of their own bodies (CPR and Bagenstos 2020). Disability groups advocated that CSCs should explicitly exempt personal ventilators belonging to chronic ventilator users from reallocation, as opposed to ventilators provided by the hospital. Many plans adopted or revised later in the pandemic reflect such protections, and the NAM (2020) statement indicates that "providers should not consider for reallocation a ventilator or other piece of life-sustaining equipment that is brought to the hospital by a patient whose life is dependent on that equipment." Individuals with disabilities have a right to bring their personal ventilators into the hospital with them as a modification to hospital policies that mandate the use of equipment only provided by hospitals—just as they have the right to bring their personal wheelchairs or hearing aids. It would be bizarre and medically counterproductive to prohibit or remove an individual's assistive technology.

How Do Crisis Standards of Care Plans Approach Disability?

Methods

As noted above, we created a dataset of 58 state CSC policies from 35 states, seeking to identify each instance of a CSC that incorporated triage of scarce treatment resources. To do so, we coded each CSC along the domains of policy variation identified above. To be included in our analysis, a policy had to be endorsed by a state agency and contain criteria for the allocation of scarce resources. State CSC policies were identified through reviews of state websites in March, August, October, and January, supplemented by existing cross-sectional reviews of state CSC policies at different points during the pandemic (Caraccio, White, and Jotwani 2020; Cleveland Manchanda, Sanky, and Appel 2020; Piscitello et al. 2020; Whyte 2020). We included only the most recent pre-pandemic CSCs in our primary analyses in tables 1–3 and figure 1 to reflect the present distribution of CSC policies as of this writing but incorporated all identified versions of a CSC issued in table 4 and figure 2 to reflect change over time.

After we identified points of variation, each author reviewed and coded relevant sections of the plans identified in our search according to an agreed-on rubric. Subsequently, the lead author conducted a secondary review and reconciled any disagreements with the initial reviewer prior to proceeding

Table 1 Summary of State CSC Plans as of January 2021 (N = 35)

	Total	
Categorical exclusions		
Incorporates	11 (31%)	
Does not incorporate	24 (69%)	
Long-term survival		
Incorporates	19 (54%)	
Does not incorporate	11 (31%)	
Does not incorporate & prohibits	5 (14%)	
Resource intensity		
Incorporates	9 (26%)	
Does not incorporate	17 (49%)	
Does not incorporate & prohibits	9 (26%)	
Reasonable modifications		
No	19 (54%)	
Yes	16 (46%)	
Chronic ventilator protections		
No	20 (57%)	
Yes	15 (43%)	
Summary Statistics for Plans by If Updated and Timing	Total	Mean disability rights index score
Never updated plans	n = 18 (51%)	1.67
Issued pre-pandemic	9 (50%)	0.78
Issued early pandemic (Feb–May 2020)	5 (28%)	1.6
Issued late pandemic (June 2020– January 2021)	4 (22%)	3.75
Updated plans	n = 17 (49%)	3.12
Last updated early pandemic (Feb–May 2020)	5 (29%)	1.67
Last updated late pandemic (June 2020–January 2021)	12 (71%)	3.43

with further analysis. Our data is available in an online-only appendix. Most coding decisions were straightforward, but the varying definitions of long- versus short-term survival required some deliberation. We ultimately chose to code a plan as incorporating long-term survival if it included allocation criteria considering survival beyond the NAM standard of "likelihood of death prior to or imminently after hospital discharge." We interpret *imminently* in this context to refer to days or weeks, not months, after hospital discharge.

For purposes of our initial analysis, we split plans into two categories reflecting whether they had been updated since their initial issuance. We constructed a Disability Rights Index Score reflecting alignment with disability rights policy preferences within a plan. The absence of exclusion criteria, the prohibition of long-term survival, the prohibition of resource intensity, the inclusion of reasonable modifications to clinical instruments, and the inclusion of chronic ventilator protections each constitute one point of five. Where CSCs do not incorporate long-term survival or resource intensity, but do not prohibit them, they receive a half point in the relevant domain. In addition, to reflect different processes of change as both advocates and policy makers developed greater expertise over the course of the pandemic, we noted the timing of plan issuance and revision and reflected two time-based categories for the purposes of subgroup analysis: early pandemic (February–May 2020) and late pandemic (June 2020–January 2021).

Results

As reflected in table 1, 18 states had not updated their plans during our review period. Of these, nine dated from prior to the pandemic, five were issued in the early pandemic, and four in the late pandemic. Seventeen states had updated their plans over the course of the pandemic, with five having most recently updated in the early period and 12 in the late period. Index scores reflect that both updated and never updated plans had higher scores in the late period.

Table 2 reflects the split between plans that were updated and those that were not along each of the five domains. Chi-squared tests are used to assess whether the presence of a revision is associated with a significant difference in the CSC domain. We find that states that revised their CSC plans are significantly more likely to lack categorical exclusions ($\chi^2(1) = 5.93$, p = 0.015) and have specified reasonable modifications ($\chi^2(1) = 4.8043$, p = 0.028). Chronic ventilator protections approach significance ($\chi^2(1) = 3.44$, p = 0.064).

Table 3 provides a subgroup analysis looking at the timing of plan revisions, using Chi-squared tests to evaluate if plans revised later in the pandemic made significantly different choices than plans revised early in the pandemic. We also reflect two-tailed t-tests comparing each domain within the early and late categories to the never updated category. We find that plans that updated late in the pandemic are less likely to have categorical exclusions ($\chi^2(1) = 5.44$, p = 0.02), more likely to prohibit or not incorporate resource intensity ($\chi^2(2) = 10.12$, p = 0.006), and more likely to specify reasonable modifications ($\chi^2(1) = 6.20$, p = 0.013) than plans updated early in the pandemic. Our t-tests also indicate that plans revised early in the pandemic were similar to those never updated, while plans

Table 2 Summary of Plans by If Updated (N = 35)

	Never updated plans n = 18	Updated plans n = 17	Total n = 35	χ^2 test
Categorical exclusions				
Incorporates	9 (50%)	2 (12%)	11 (31%)	
Does not incorporate	9 (50%)	15 (88%)	24 (69%)	(1) = 5.93, p = 0.015*
Long-term survival				
Incorporates	11 (61%)	8 (47%)	19 (54%)	
Does not incorporate	6 (33%)	5 (29%)	11 (31%)	
Does not incorporate & prohibits	1 (6%)	4 (24%)	5 (14%)	(2) = 2.34, p = 0.311
Resource intensity				
Incorporates	6 (33%)	3 (18%)	9 (26%)	
Does not incorporate	10 (56%)	7 (41%)	17 (49%)	
Does not incorporate & prohibits	2 (11%)	7 (41%)	9 (26%)	(2) = 4.28, p = 0.118
Reasonable modifications				
No	13 (72%)	6 (35%)	19 (54%)	
Yes	5 (28%)	11 (65%)	16 (46%)	(1) = 4.8043, p = 0.028*
Chronic ventilator protections				
No	13 (72%)	7 (41%)	20 (57%)	
Yes	5 (28%)	10 (59%)	15 (43%)	(1) = 3.44, p = 0.064

Note: Column percentages for each category are reported in parentheses. Percentages may not total 100 due to rounding. * p < 0.05, ** p < 0.01, *** p < 0.001.

Table 3 Timing of CSC Plan Changes

	Last update early in pandemic (February–May 2020) n = 5	Last update later in the pandemic (June 2020–January 2021) n = 12	Total	χ^2 test comparing early and late
Categorical exclusions				
Incorporates	2 (40%) [p = 0.717]	0 (0%)*** [p < 0.000]	2 (12%)	(1) = 5.44, p = 0.02*
Does not incorporate	3 (60%) [p = 0.717]	12 (100%)*** [p < 0.000]	15 (88%)	
Long-term survival				
Incorporates	3 (60%) [p = 0.968]	5 (42%) [p = 0.313]	8 (47%)	(2) = 2.19, p = 0.335
Does not incorporate	2 (40%) [p = 0.807]	3 (25%) [p = 0.634]	5 (29%)	
Does not incorporate & prohibits	0 (0%) [p = 0.324]	4 (33%) [p = 0.078]	4 (24%)	
Resource intensity				
Incorporates	3 (60%) [p = 0.331]	0 (0%)** [p = 0.006]	3 (18%)	(2) = 10.12, p = 0.006**
Does not incorporate	2 (40%) [p = 0.573]	5 (42%) [p = 0.473]	7 (41%)	
Does not incorporate & prohibits	0 (0%) [p = 0.154]	7 (58%)** [p = 0.008]	7 (58%)	

(continued)

Table 3 Timing of CSC Plan Changes (*continued*)

	Last update early in pandemic (February–May 2020) n = 5	Last update later in the pandemic (June 2020–January 2021) n = 12	Total	χ² test comparing early and late
Reasonable modifications				
No	4 (80%) [p=0.735]	2 (17%)*** [p=0.001]	6 (35%)	
Yes	1 (20%) [p=0.735]	10 (83%)*** [p=0.001]	11 (65%)	(1)=6.20, p=0.013*
Chronic ventilator protections				
No	3 (60%) [p=0.651]	4 (33%)* [p=0.037]	7 (41%)	
Yes	2 (40%) [p=0.651]	8 (67%)* [p=0.037]	10 (59%)	(1)=1.04, p=0.309

Note: p-values reflect t-tests for difference from the unchanged plan category. Chi-squared tests reflect differences between early and late pandemic. * p<0.05, ** p<0.01, *** p<0.001.

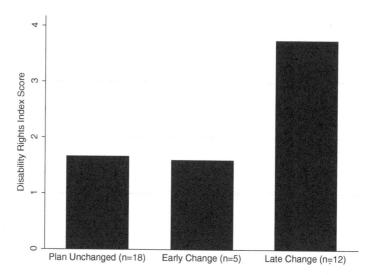

Figure 1   Mean disability rights index score by if updated and update timing.

updated late in the pandemic were different from those never updated on every domain except long-term survival. Figure 1 reflects this graphically using our constructed Disability Rights Index Score.

We also reviewed within-state variation by reviewing 23 state plan revisions within 17 states (table 4). With the exception of New Mexico, Arizona, and Alabama adding long-term survival, and Vermont's addition of categorical exclusions, all other revisions were toward greater alignment with disability rights priorities. We also reflect index scores for each new state plan and revision in order of release in figure 2, which reflects a shift toward greater alignment with disability rights priorities over the course of the pandemic.

Limitations

While our analysis compares states that never updated their CSCs to those that did, some states in the former group issued CSCs relatively late in the pandemic and were thus exposed to models and activist pressure that early states were not. The inclusion of early and late never-updated states in the same category may mean that we understate the extent of CSC policy evolution by using both early and late never-updated plans as a point of comparison with updated plans. To address this, we provide analyses showing change over time across all plans in the online-only appendix. These reflect

Table 4 Changes within States during the Pandemic as of January 2021

Greater Alignment with Disability Rights Positions

	Exclusions added	Exclusions removed	
Categorical exclusions (8 modifications)	1	7	

	Provision added	Provision removed	Prohibited
Long-term survival (12 modifications)	3	5	4
Resource intensity (11 modifications)	0	4	7

	Protection removed	Protection added	
Reasonable modifications (11 modifications)	0	11	
Chronic ventilator protections (11 modifications)	0	11	

Note: Where plans were withdrawn without immediate replacement and included one of the provisions in question, we reflect this as removal.

similar results showing greater alignment with disability rights priorities over time, beginning from a worse pre-pandemic baseline.

While coding was relatively straightforward across most of our domains, determining how to code long-term survival in state CSC plans presented some difficult choices. States have defined short- and long-term survival differently. We chose a conservative approach, interpreting the NAM's standard of "likelihood of death prior to or imminently after hospital discharge" as referring to a window of days or at most weeks after discharge, not months. We did so because we believe it is the appropriate standard. However, by sweeping both 10-year and 6-month survival windows into the same category, significant policy change within this domain likely went undetected.

We also note that some points of policy variation emerged too late to be included in our analysis. A growing number of states have adopted CSC provisions requested by disability groups designed to ensure that patients are not "steered" or pressured into consenting to the denial or withdrawal of life-sustaining care, including through advanced care planning decisions.

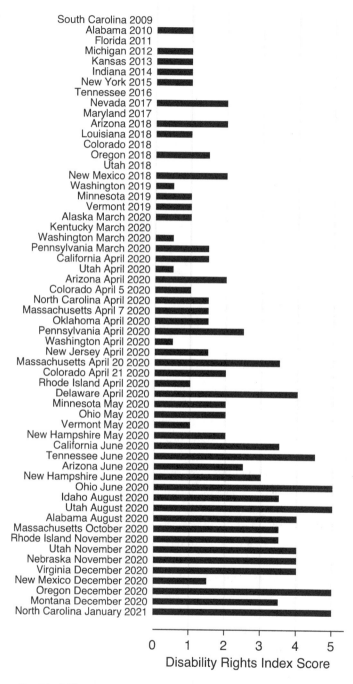

Figure 2 Disability rights index scores over time.

This is an important area of both CSC and general end-of-life policy variation that we intend to explore in future work.

Some states have declined to issue CSCs, deferring to hospital systems and other providers to develop their own plans, a level of variation that our analysis does not capture. Finally, while we identified CSCs issued through January 2021, CSC policy is still evolving and we anticipate that further CSCs are likely to be issued that we do not capture.

Venue Shopping, Competing Frames, and Bioethics Policy Change

Disability advocates have made significant progress in advancing their policy positions over the course of the pandemic, with the notable exception of long-term survival, which continues to be a source of concern for disability and racial justice activists. Our findings show that CSC plans revised later in the pandemic were more likely to align with disability rights priorities than those revised early in the pandemic or never revised. This pattern is consistent with growth over time in both the familiarity of state policy makers with disability rights concerns and the capacity of disability activists to influence public policy on a topic that has quickly moved from obscurity to prominence.

Disability advocates pursued a variety of avenues for advancing CSC policy changes. The website of the Center for Public Representation (CPR 2021), a disability group at the center of CSC advocacy nationally, references letters from advocates in 38 states and more than a dozen legal complaints. While some state plans describe collaborative processes through which policy makers and activists mediated disputes, negotiations took place against a backdrop of unprecedented advocacy mobilization and media interest in medical rationing, empowering activists to win victories that would not have been possible prior to the pandemic.

This raises important questions about the process of change in bioethics policy making. While much has been written about the merits of different CSC approaches (Bagenstos 2020; Emanuel et al. 2020; Ne'eman 2020; Persad 2020), little research has examined the processes by which they evolve over time. This is somewhat surprising. Though many CSC plans were influential at the start of the emergency, the extent to which nearly two decades of clinician-led CSC policy development proved of limited relevance as COVID-19 continued is genuinely shocking. Ideas that were considered central to CSC policy making prior to the pandemic, such as the use of exclusion criteria and resource-intensity judgments, have been removed and in some instances prohibited from use based on civil rights concerns. While many CSCs adopted early or pre-pandemic do not yet reflect this progress, the December NAM statement reflected a major shift, endorsing disability-rights CSC priorities across the board. Though it may take some time for this progress to be consolidated across the country, the direction of policy making has changed dramatically. Exploring why may yield important insights on the nature of bioethics policy change more generally. Though we do not document the explicit process that led to CSC policy evolution in this article, the direction of these changes and the context within which they took place allow us to offer some suggestive hypotheses to help inform future work.

One potential explanation may simply be greater visibility. Pre–COVID-19 CSC policy debates did not attract the same level of mobilization. Even when activists were aware of CSC policy making and chose to devote scarce resources to a hypothetical threat, they were unlikely to have the same influence before COVID-19 placed CSCs in the media spotlight. Given the exigencies of COVID-19, clinicians are likely displaying more flexibility than they would have previously, as the need for regulatory certainty in a crisis may be more important than a preferred policy arrangement.

Whatever the reason, CSC policy making has witnessed a rapid evolution from an expert-led process rooted in the norms of clinical and academic bioethics to an arena in which clinicians and consumer stakeholders must mediate their disputes on a somewhat more equal playing field. While clinicians still have a central role in CSC policy making, they are now as likely to sit across from civil rights lawyers as they are moral philosophers. The venue of debate has changed, possibly permanently.

The political science literature has much to say about such transitions. Building on Robert A. Dahl's conception of a pluralist government made up of multiple overlapping but distinct domains of policy-making authority, Frank Baumgartner and Bryan Jones (1991) explored the process of "venue shopping" used by both industry and activist stakeholders to achieve a more favorable reception for their policy views. Such venue shopping seeks to "alter the roster of participants who are involved in the issue" by framing it as within the province of policy makers friendly to each side's priorities.

Baumgartner and Jones note that under pluralist arrangements industries may "insulate themselves from the influence of large-scale democratic forces through the creation of relatively independent depoliticized subgovernments" (1045). As an issue becomes more controversial, politicization ensues and the possibility of a change in venue becomes more plausible. They elaborate:

Technically complex issues . . . can be discussed either in terms of their scientific . . . details, or in terms of their social impacts. When they are portrayed as technical problems rather than as social questions, experts can dominate the decision-making process. When the ethical, social or political implications of such policies assume center stage, a much broader range of participants can suddenly become involved. Where a positive image dominates, specialists have strong arguments for demanding that political leaders grant them . . . autonomy. (1047)

However, when that positive image changes—perhaps as a result of increased public scrutiny in a crisis—an opportunity to shift venues and broaden the range of participants emerges.

Bioethics debates are uniquely well situated for venue shopping, as they cross multiple disciplines. It is rarely clear what policy makers have final responsibility for or which experts are most qualified to opine in bioethics disputes, not least because their typical combination of obscurity and controversy may not lend themselves to enthusiastic claims of ownership. Activists and providers who disagree on the substance of bioethics debates may play out such disagreements in part through disputes about which government agency or professional discipline has authority over them. Tensions between the civil rights and clinical frames to CSC policy may be best understood through this lens.

While it is certainly possible that the end of the public health emergency will mean a return to the status quo, it seems unlikely. Activists have built capacity that will persist. In the near term, it will likely be deployed to other COVID-19 priorities, such as vaccine allocation. In the long term, it may be used to address bioethics controversies unrelated to the pandemic, such as disputes about qualitative futility judgments or QALY-based rationing. Anthony Downs (1972) noted that issues that capture the public imagination are usually permanently changed, even after the public's attention moves elsewhere.

It is worth considering the rationale behind this venue shift and its implications for policy makers. With some exceptions (such as abortion), policy on controversial bioethics issues has usually been shaped by expert judgment, with legislators providing broad deference to clinicians and bioethicists to police their own behavior. Nominally, this is because of superior expertise to answer complex questions. But complexity is not the only factor that drives delegation.

Others have noted the risk that expert delegation may limit democratic accountability in the context of legislative delegation to executive branch bureaucracies (Fox and Jordan 2011). Bioethics policy decisions involve a similar form of delegation, from traditional policy makers to experts in academia and medicine. As with congressional delegation, this can offer a mechanism to avoid controversial policy decisions. While complexity means some delegation is necessary, excess delegation is concerning.

Elected officials, appointees, and even civil servants are more likely to be responsive to stakeholder activism emphasizing the distributive consequences of bioethics policy. Delegation to experts deprives marginalized groups of an effective means of influencing policy that impacts their lives. Some maintain that this reduced democratic accountability is a positive feature, not a flaw, as it allows for more impartial, technocratic decision making by the bioethics profession. According to this thinking, resolving bioethics disputes via the political process fails to adequately represent the interests of those who are unaware they are at risk "while protecting the interests of a small group that is better positioned to organize" (Persad 2020: 48).

This argument might carry more weight if policy makers could delegate to truly impartial arbiters able to weigh the consequences of every policy choice without bias or self-interest. But in the real world, we must remember that clinical bioethics is not simply a field of intellectual inquiry. It is also a professional discipline with a distinct worldview and biases inherited from the medical profession and the broader society, which shape bioethicist views on disability (Iezzoni et al. 2021; Stramondo 2021). As Gregor Wolbring (2003) notes, mainstream bioethics often finds itself unsympathetic to disability rights claims in part because the field's grounding in a medical framework primes its members to see disability only in medical terms, rather than the disability rights movement's preferred civil rights frame (a distinction that reaffirms the importance of venue shopping in bioethics policy disputes). It should be noted that the field of bioethics is not a monolith. In part because of the aforementioned shortcomings, recent years have seen the emergence of a "disability bioethics," informed by the disability rights movement's values framework and the lived experiences of disabled people, intended to serve as a counter to more traditional "mainstream bioethics" (Stramondo 2021; Wolbring 2003). Analogous to similar feminist bioethics critiques, disability bioethics is deployed by its proponents to challenge the perceived excesses and errors of mainstream bioethics practice and to promote a civil rights frame in relevant discussions of bioethics disputes regarding disability.

In addition, because mainstream clinical bioethicists make decisions that can expose them and the providers that often employ them to legal risk, they are incentivized to shape public policy to minimize liability. Policy positions advanced from this sector thus cannot be viewed as intellectual abstractions but must also be considered within the context of a profession that seeks to shape its own regulatory constraints. To be clear, bioethicists from many different backgrounds have much to contribute to policy debates through their specialized expertise—but the close relationship and overlap between mainstream clinical bioethicists and the broader medical profession means that policy makers should understand their advice as that of an interested stakeholder, akin to a labor union or industry group. Respect for professional expertise of those a policy maker is regulating is important—but absolute deference is inappropriate.

From this perspective, mainstream bioethicists should be seen as one stakeholder among many at policy tables convened to mediate bioethics disputes, rather than as the chair or convener. Policy makers should see themselves as mediators between a profession that offers substantive expertise but desires to minimize liability and consumer stakeholders that seek greater regulatory oversight to protect against discrimination. This is a not unfamiliar dynamic, similar to many other instances in which policy makers must mediate between industry and consumer stakeholders. While more difficult, policy-maker mediation is superior to expert delegation, for it offers a more transparent and accountable process with a greater likelihood of accounting for distributional consequences to marginalized groups.

The unprecedented public visibility given to CSCs as a result of the COVID-19 pandemic may have begun such process shifts, prompting a "change of venue" for bioethics policy making, but they are unlikely to end there. Policy makers that may have previously seen delegation to experts as a safe avenue for avoiding responsibility for difficult choices found themselves facing public backlash and potential legal liability for the CSCs they had previously endorsed. Deference to expert judgment on resource allocation will no longer seem the safe option it once was, even post–COVID-19. We theorize that when public backlash mitigates the political benefit of expert delegation, policy makers are more willing to directly mediate policy disputes between experts and consumer stakeholders, resulting in policy changes more closely aligned with the latter's views.

While further research is necessary to validate these ideas, the process of change in state CSCs is consistent with them. Categorical exclusions, the most visible form of disability discrimination, were quickly removed from existing plans and left out of most new ones as media attention increased during the early phase of the pandemic, even though they had been central to pre-pandemic CSC planning. Other disability rights priorities, such as prohibiting prioritization based on resource intensity and requiring reasonable modifications, were more common in plans issued later in the pandemic, after stakeholder groups developed greater expertise to influence policy makers. Regardless, CSC revisions regarding disability were almost always in favor of greater alignment with disability rights positions, suggesting that stakeholder engagement proved an effective avenue for modifying policies that were previously the exclusive domain of experts.

Subsequent inquiries should more closely examine public opinion and the process of bioethics policy change at the micro-level, looking closely at different venues for debate. Various experimental methods, such as conjoint analysis, may help explain the salience of different diagnoses and their intersection with other forms of marginalized identity.

COVID-19 has provided a vivid illustration of the stakes of bioethics policy. Our review suggests that the disability rights movement has had increasing success in influencing CSC policy as the pandemic has proceeded, though some of this influence is not yet reflected in plans that have not been recently updated. Further research should explore the process of bioethics decision making and the ways in which experts and other stakeholders conflict and collaborate in shaping policy.

■ ■ ■

Ari Ne'eman is a PhD candidate in health policy at Harvard University. He is a senior research associate at the Harvard Law School Project on Disability and a visiting scholar at the Lurie Institute for Disability Policy at Brandeis University. He cofounded the Autistic Self Advocacy Network and served as its executive director from 2006 to 2016. He also served as one of President Obama's appointees to the National Council on Disability from 2010 to 2015.
aneeman@g.harvard.edu

Michael Ashley Stein is the executive director of the Harvard Law School Project on Disability, a visiting professor at Harvard Law School, and an extraordinary professor at the University of Pretoria Faculty of Law Centre for Human Rights.

Zackary D. Berger is an associate professor at the Johns Hopkins School of Medicine and a member of the core faculty at the Johns Hopkins Berman Institute of Bioethics. He also holds a joint appointment at the Johns Hopkins Bloomberg School of Public Health. He has conducted ethics consultation for, and treated, COVID-19 in the inpatient and outpatient settings.

Doron Dorfman is an associate professor of law at the Syracuse University College of Law and a member of the SUNY Upstate Medical University Bioethics Committee. He is also a faculty affiliate with the Disability Law and Policy Program as well the Aging Studies Institute at Syracuse University.

Acknowledgments

The authors wish to thank Kit Albrecht, the editors of *JHPPL*, and two anonymous peer reviewers for their helpful feedback in the development of this piece. Research reported in this publication was supported by the National Institute of Mental Health of the National Institutes of Health under award number T32MH019733. The content is solely the responsibility of the authors and does not necessarily represent the official views of the National Institutes of Health. Mr. Ne'eman reports consulting income within the last three years from the American Civil Liberties Union, the Partnership to Improve Patient Care, and the Department of Health and Human Services Office of Civil Rights. The data presented here was not collected as part of his duties for any of these entities, including the Department of Health and Human Services, and the research, analysis, findings, and conclusions were not reviewed by them nor do they necessarily represent their views.

References

ASTP (American Society for Transplant Physicians). 1998. "International Guidelines for the Selection of Lung Transplant Candidates." *American Journal of Respiratory and Critical Care Medicine* 158, no. 1: 335–39. doi.org/10.1164/ajrccm.158.1.15812.

Bagenstos, Samuel. 2009. *Law and the Contradictions of the Disability Rights Movement.* New Haven, CT: Yale University Press.

Bagenstos, Samuel. 2020. "Who Gets the Ventilator? Disability Discrimination in COVID-19 Medical-Rationing Protocols." *Yale Law Journal* 130: 1–25. www.yalelawjournal.org/forum/who-gets-the-ventilator.

Bateman, Scot, Paul Biddinger, Cheri Blauwet, Peter DePergola II, Deb Enos, Lachlan Forrow, Eric Goralnick, et al. 2020. "Crisis Standard of Care Planning Guidance for the COVID-19 Pandemic." Department of Public Health, Executive Office of Health and Human Services, Commonwealth of Massachusetts, April 7 (revised October 20). www.mass.gov/doc/crisis-standards-of-care-planning-guidance-for-the-covid-19-pandemic/download.

Baumgartner, Frank, and Bryan Jones. 1991. "Agenda Dynamics and Policy Subsystems." *Journal of Politics* 53, no. 4: 1044–74.

Brown, Matthew J., and Justin Goodwin. 2020. "Correspondence: Allocating Medical Resources in the Time of Covid-19." *New England Journal of Medicine* 382, no. 22: e79. doi.org/10.1056/NEJMc2009666.

Caraccio, Caiara, Robert S. White, and Rohan Jotwani. 2020. "No Protocol and No Liability: A Call for COVID Crisis Guidelines That Protect Vulnerable Populations." *Journal of Comparative Effectiveness Research* 9, no. 12: 829–37. doi.org/10.2217/cer-2020-0090.

Christian, Michael D., Laura Hawryluck, Randy S. Wax, Tim Cook, Neil M. Lazar, Margaret S. Herridge, Matthew P. Muller, Douglas R. Gowans, Wendy Fortier, and Frederick M. Burkle. 2006. "Development of a Triage Protocol for Critical Care during an Influenza Pandemic." *Canadian Medical Association Journal* 175, no. 11: 1377–81. doi.org/10.1503/cmaj.060911.

Cleveland Manchanda, Emily C., Charles Sanky, and Jacob M. Appel. 2020. "Crisis Standards of Care in the USA: A Systematic Review and Implications for Equity amidst COVID-19." *Journal of Racial and Ethnic Health Disparities*, August 13. doi.org/10.1007/s40615-020-00840-5.

CPR (Center for Public Representation). 2021. "COVID-19 Medical Rationing and Facility Visitation Policies." January 15. www.centerforpublicrep.org/covid-19-medical-rationing/.

CPR (Center for Public Representation) and Sam Bagenstos. 2020. "Evaluation Framework for Crisis Standard of Care Plans." April 9 (updated November 30). www.centerforpublicrep.org/wp-content/uploads/Updated-evaluation-framework.pdf.

Downs, Anthony. 1972. "Up and Down with Ecology—the 'Issue-Attention Cycle.'" *Public Interest* 28: 38–50.

Emanuel, Ezekiel J., Govind Persad, Ross Upshur, Beatriz Thome, Michael Parker, Aaron Glickman, Cathy Zhang, Connor Boyle, Maxwell Smith, and James P. Phillips. 2020. "Fair Allocation of Scarce Medical Resources in the Time of Covid-19." *New England Journal of Medicine* 382, no. 21: 2049–55. doi.org/10.1056/NEJMsb2005114.

Fox, Justin, and Stuart V. Jordan. 2011. "Delegation and Accountability." *Journal of Politics* 73, no. 3: 831–44. doi.org/10.1017/s0022381611000491.

Francis, Leslie, and Anita Silvers. 2017. "Reading Alexander V. Choate Rightly: Now Is the Time." *Laws* 6, no. 4. doi.org/10.3390/laws6040017.

Iezzoni, Lisa I., Sowmya R. Rao, Julie Ressalam, Dragana Bolcic-Jankovic, Nicole D. Agaronnik, Karen Donelan, Tara Lagu, and Eric G. Campbell. 2021. "Physicians' Perceptions of People with Disability and Their Health Care." *Health Affairs* 40, no. 2: 297–306. doi.org/10.1377/hlthaff.2020.01452.

IOM (Institute of Medicine). 2009. "Crisis Standards of Care: The Vision." In *Guidance for Establishing Crisis Standards of Care for Use in Disaster Situations: A Letter Report*, edited by Bruce M. Altevogt, Clare Stroud, Sarah L. Hanson, Dan Hanfling, and Lawrence O. Gostin, 17–22. Washington, DC: National Academies Press.

Kerem, Eitan, Joseph Reisman, Mary Corey, Gerard J. Canny, and Henry Levison. 1992. "Prediction of Mortality in Patients with Cystic Fibrosis." *New England Journal of Medicine* 326, no. 18: 1187–91. doi.org/10.1056/NEJM199204303261804.

Krahn, Gloria L., Deborah Klein Walker, and Rosaly Correa-De-Araujo. 2015. "Persons with Disabilities as an Unrecognized Health Disparity Population." *American Journal of Public Health* 105, no. S2: S198–S206. doi.org/10.2105/AJPH.2014.302182.

Milla, Carlos E., and Warren J. Warwick. 1998. "Risk of Death in Cystic Fibrosis Patients with Severely Compromised Lung Function." *Chest* 113, no. 5: 1230–34. doi.org/10.1378/chest.113.5.1230.

NAM (National Academy of Medicine). 2020. "National Organizations Call for Action to Implement Crisis Standards of Care during COVID-19 Surge." December 18. nam.edu/national-organizations-call-for-action-to-implement-crisis-standards -of-care-during-covid-19-surge/.

NCD (National Council on Disability). 2019. "Bioethics and Disability Report Series." September 25–November 20. ncd.gov/publications/2019/bioethics-report-series.

Ne'eman, Ari. 2020. "When It Comes to Rationing, Disability Rights Law Prohibits More than Prejudice." Hastings Center, April 10. www.thehastingscenter.org/when -it-comes-to-rationing-disability-rights-law-prohibits-more-than-prejudice/.

Network for Public Health Law. 2020. "COVID-19: Racial Disparities and Crisis Standards of Care." May. www.networkforphl.org/wp-content/uploads/2020/05 /COVID-19-Racial-Disparities-and-Crisis-Standards-of-Care.pdf.

Pendo, Elizabeth. 2020. "COVID-19 and Disability-Based Discrimination in Health Care." American Bar Association, May 22. www.americanbar.org/groups/diversity /disabilityrights/resources/covid19-disability-discrimination/.

Persad, Govind. 2020. "Disability Law and the Case for Evidence-Based Triage in a Pandemic." *Yale Law Journal* 130: 26–50.

Piscitello, Gina M., Esha M. Kapania, William D. Miller, Juan C. Rojas, Mark Siegler, and William F. Parker. 2020. "Variation in Ventilator Allocation Guidelines by US State during the Coronavirus Disease 2019 Pandemic: A Systematic Review." *JAMA Network Open* 3, no. 6: e2012606. doi.org/10.1001/jamanetworkopen.2020.12606.

Pressley, Ayanna. 2020. "Rep. Pressley Calls on Governor Baker to Rescind Crisis of Care Standards That Disproportionately Harm Communities of Color and Disability Community." Press release, April 13. pressley.house.gov/media/press-releases/rep -pressley-calls-governor-baker-rescind-crisis-care-standards.

RIDOH (Rhode Island Department of Health). 2020. "Crisis Standards of Care Guidelines." December 4. health.ri.gov/publications/guidelines/crisis-standards -of-care.pdf.

Schmidt, Harald, Dorothy E. Roberts, and Nwamaka D. Eneanya. 2021. "Rationing, Racism, and Justice: Advancing the Debate around 'Colourblind' COVID-19 Ventilator Allocation." *Journal of Medical Ethics*, January 6. doi.org/10.1136/medethics-2020-106856.

Stein, Michael Ashley. 2003. "The Law and Economics of Disability Accommodations." *Duke Law Journal* 53, no. 1: 79–191.

Stein, Michael Ashley, and Michael E. Waterstone. 2006. "Disability, Disparate Impact, and Class Actions." *Duke Law Journal* 56, no. 3: 861–922.

Stramondo, Joseph A. 2020. "Disability, Likelihood of Survival, and Inefficiency amidst Pandemic." April 6. www.bioethics.net/2020/04/disability-likelihood-of -survival-and-inefficiency-amidst-pandemic/.

Stramondo, Joseph A. 2021. "Bioethics, Adaptive Preferences, and Judging the Quality of a Life with Disability." *Social Theory and Practice* 47, no. 1: 199–220. doi.org/ 10.5840/soctheorpract202121117.

Wasserman, David, Govind Persad, and Joseph Millum. 2020. "Setting Priorities Fairly in Response to Covid-19: Identifying Overlapping Consensus and Reasonable Disagreement." *Journal of Law and the Biosciences* 7, no. 1: 1–12. academic.oup.com/jlb/article/7/1/lsaa044/5862544.

Whyte, Liz Essley. 2020. "State Policies May Send People with Disabilities to the Back of the Line for Ventilators." Center for Public Integrity, April 8. publicintegrity.org/health/coronavirus-and-inequality/state-policies-may-send-people-with-disabilities-to-the-back-of-the-line-for-ventilators/.

Wolbring, Gregor. 2003. "Disability Rights Approach toward Bioethics?" *Journal of Disability Policy Studies* 14, no. 3: 174–80.

Compounding Racialized Vulnerability: COVID-19 in Prisons, Jails, and Migrant Detention Centers

Matthew G. T. Denney
Ramon Garibaldo Valdez
Yale University

Abstract

Context: Carceral institutions are among the largest clusters of COVID-19 in the United States. In response, activists and detainees have rallied around decarceration demands: the release of detainees and inmates to prevent exposure to COVID-19. This article theorizes the compounding racial vulnerability that has led to such a marked spread behind bars, mainly among race-class subjugated (RCS) communities.

Methods: The authors provide an in-depth account of COVID-19 in American correctional facilities and the mobilization to reduce contagions. They also use two survey experiments to describe public support for harm reduction and decarceration demands and to measure the effects of information about racial inequalities in prison and poor conditions inside migrant detention centers.

Findings: The authors found only one-third to one-half of respondents believe that response to COVID-19 in prisons and immigrant detention centers should be a high priority. They also found Americans are more supportive of harm reduction measures than decarceration efforts. Information about racial disparities increases support decarceration. They did not find any significant effect of information about poor conditions in migrant detention centers.

Conclusions: The conditions in carceral institutions during the pandemic—and public opinion about them—highlight the realities of compounding racialized vulnerability in the United States.

Keywords COVID-19, criminal justice, health disparities, systemic racism, public opinion

> Racism, specifically, is the state-sanctioned or extralegal production and exploitation of group-differentiated vulnerability to premature death.
> —Ruth Wilson Gilmore, *Golden Gulag: Prison, Surplus, Crisis, and Opposition in Globalizing California*

Journal of Health Politics, Policy and Law, Vol. 46, No. 5, October 2021
DOI 10.1215/03616878-9156019 © 2021 by Duke University Press

Crisis and Resistance in San Quentin State Prison

Christopher Hickson tested positive for COVID-19 on a Saturday morning. "I felt devastated. I have watched on television and read about it. I feared for my life because of how many precious lives this virus has taken," said Hickson in an interview. It was June 27, 2020, when a guard notified him of his status and instructed him to remain in his cell (Moreno Haines 2020). Later that day, Hickson and 60 other COVID-19–positive prisoners in San Quentin State Prison in California were moved to Badger Section, where they were forced to withstand isolation without cleaning supplies or electrical power. Hickson and 19 other prisoners launched a hunger strike to draw attention to their plight. The group demanded improved conditions in Badger Section and in San Quentin as a whole as well as a halt to all transfers between and inside California prisons. They claimed that, rather than containing the virus, shifting COVID-19–positive individuals between facilities simply guaranteed its spread (Moreno Haines 2020).

Available data backs the assessment of the hunger strikers. San Quentin had managed to remain free of COVID-19 until May 30, when 121 people were transferred from the California Institution for Men in Chino (Moreno Haines and Weil-Greenberg 2020). At the peak of San Quentin's pandemic, 1,636 prisoners—one-third of the prison's population—were COVID-19 positive and 72 of them had died (Clayton 2020). In a matter of days, San Quentin became the largest cluster of COVID-19 in the country (*New York Times* 2020). The hunger strikers were not merely denouncing the conditions at Badger Section: they were putting forth an analysis of a growing crisis across the country. The story of San Quentin—the protest of those inside, the reticence of the administration, the harrowing effects of COVID-19—mirrors the tragedy inside countless prisons, detention centers, and jails across the United States. According to data from the Marshall Project (2020), as of January 28, there have been more than 365,924 cases of COVID-19 and 2,314 deaths reported in carceral institutions. The five largest US clusters of COVID-19 since the outbreak of the pandemic have been correctional institutions (Williams, Seline, and Griesbach 2020). It seemed, however, that the American public had either forgotten about the people behind bars or, worse, accepted the inevitability of their suffering and death.

The COVID-19 crisis behind bars is one whose roots lay within America's twin crises of mass incarceration and structural racism. In this article, we seek to illuminate the compounding racial vulnerability brought by COVID-19 to carceral institutions. The first part clarifies the significance of racialized vulnerability in the United States, and it identifies how patterns of systematic racism set the stage for disproportionate exposure to harm during the COVID-19 crisis. The second part provides an in-depth account of the harm done by COVID-19 inside jails, prisons, and immigrant detention centers. Consequently, it outlines the policy demands expressed by advocates both inside and outside prisons. The third part describes public opinion on COVID-19 in prisons and migrant detention centers. Our two survey experiments were fielded in the early spring—prior to the wave of racial justice protests—measuring support for the policies pushed by advocates. We exposed some of our respondents to informational treatments about racial inequities in prisons and poor conditions inside immigrant detention centers. We argue that our survey findings demonstrate public indifference toward the spread of COVID-19 in prisons. Though awareness of racial injustice may bring greater attention to the crisis, it is not enough to address the racial vulnerability faced by affected populations.

Theory and Background: Racism as Exposure to Premature Death

In this article we put forth the notion of "compounding racial vulnerability" to describe the disproportionate effects of external shocks, such as COVID-19, on race-class subjugated (RCS) communities. We argue that public health crises are exacerbated among RCS communities because of the arrangements of structural racism and by governmental responses to the crisis. Our conceptualization of compounding racial vulnerability has three elements: (1) the existence of health care inequities along lines of race and class, (2) an external shock that disproportionately affects RCS communities, and (3) a governmental response that heightens the unequal impact of the shock. We argue that the disproportionate spread of COVID-19 in carceral institutions is caused by the existing inequities of structural racism. These structures are in part sustained by public opinion and public preferences along the proverbial "color line" (Du Bois [1903] 2003) of race. Our survey analysis reveals a disregard for the welfare of inmates—who mostly come from RCS communities—and a lack of political will to address the causes of the crisis, mostly among white Americans but still present to a lesser degree among nonwhites.

Our surveys also show that public indifference may be ameliorated with information about unequal racial outcomes in the criminal justice system, though not enough to prompt our respondents to prioritize COVID-19 preventive measures behind bars, support decarceration, or address the systemic roots of the crisis. The theoretical contributions made by this article are also in line with other analyses of structural racism in the context of COVID-19 (Pirtle 2020; Sewell 2020). Furthermore, we believe the notion of compounding racial vulnerability describes the consequences of other disasters among RCSs; one example other than COVID-19 may be found in the government's and the public's response to Hurricane Katrina in New Orleans. As was the case with COVID-19, Katrina largely affected the Black community, and its impact was made worse by the racially unequal distribution of resources in the city and the political indifference of government agencies (BondGraham 2007; Frymer, Strolovitch, and Warren 2006; Stivers 2007).

Understanding the impact of COVID-19 in carceral institutions and public opinion requires placing the pandemic within America's larger context of structural racism, "the totality of ways in which societies foster racial discrimination through mutually reinforcing systems of housing, education, employment, earning, benefits, credit, media, health care, and criminal justice" (Bailey et al. 2017: 1453). In contrast to the view that racism is limited to ideational prejudices or to the remnants of pre-1965 de jure segregation, the notion of structural racism describes resource and power inequities consistently perpetuated along lines of race (Bonilla-Silva 1997; Omi and Winant 2015). Bailey and coauthors (2017) argue that a theoretical focus on structural racism explains persistent inequities in public health outcomes through myriad pathways, including environmental health (e.g., the lack of drinking water in Flint, Michigan), psychosocial trauma, targeted marketing of health-harming substances, inadequate health care, maladaptive coping behaviors, and stereotype threats.

One of the most radical expressions of structural racism is the centrality of the criminal justice system to the lives of nonwhite communities in the United States. To describe the importance of both structural racism and capitalism, Joe Soss and Vesla Weaver (2017) coined the term *race-class subjugated communities* (RCS). These communities, they argue, are politically characterized not as formal actors in government institutions but as targets of state policies. Rather than alleviate inequities, state actors perpetuate them through practices of "coercion, containment, repression, surveillance, regulation, predation, discipline, and violence" (567).

Law enforcement agencies have been key actors in the American systematization of racism (Hadden 2003). These patterns have evolved over time into the present era of mass criminalization (Gottschalk 2015; Lerman and Weaver 2014; Western 2006). Incarceration and policing are employed in the United States to respond to the very conditions of poverty and unrest prompted by structural racism; in return, criminalization has worsened the inequalities it is meant to address (Alexander 2010; Western 2006). As the criminal justice system has expanded, it has also worsened the social vulnerability of migrant populations (Macias-Rojas 2016). Since the late 1990s, immigration and criminal justice policies have taken a punitive turn through local-federal enforcement collaborations (e.g., the Secure Communities [S-Comm] program), increased deportations, and increased migrant detention (Golash-Boza 2015; Lopez 2019; Sampaio 2015).

One need not look behind bars to see the disproportionate impact of COVID-19 on race-class subjugated communities. Data from the Color of Coronavirus Project (collected mid-March 2020 through February 4, 2021) shows an age-adjusted COVID-19 mortality rate among Blacks, Latinxs, and Native Americans twice as high as that among white people. At one point (October 13, 2020), the rate among Native Americans was three times as high as that of white Americans. Nationwide, Black Americans represent 15.7% of all deaths of known race despite being 12.4% of the population. For their part, Latino Americans have experienced 18.1% of all deaths of known race and represent 16.3% of the population (APM Research Lab 2020). These racial disparities have also been present in vaccination rates. Data from the CDC (2021) shows that as of February 26, 2021, 64.4% of those vaccinated are non-Hispanic white, while only 8.7% are Latino and 6.5% are Black.

Jose F. Figueroa and colleagues (2020) find that in the state of Massachusetts, "independent predictors of higher COVID-19 rates include the proportion of foreign-born noncitizens living in a community, mean household size, and share of food service workers." Nonwhites are more likely to work in occupational sectors keeping them in close contact with others (Oppel et al. 2020). High residential density has also led to a quicker spread of COVID-19 among RCS: "Latino people are twice as likely to reside in a crowded dwelling—less than 500 square feet per person—as white people, according to the American Housing Survey" (Oppel et al. 2020). Resource scarcity and preexisting health issues have worsened the pandemic in areas highly populated by RCS communities, such as the Southern borderlands or Indian Country (Dickerson 2020; Walker 2020).

On top of a virus that has exacerbated structural vulnerability, governmental responses have either disregarded or harmed RCS communities. The federal government pushed for a speedy reopening of the economy and more lax public health measures merely months into the crisis, even as the contagion and death rate among Black Americans and other people of color rose (Adamy 2020). These inequalities, and the government's disregard, were made evident during the racial justice protests that ensued in the summer of 2020 and were widely met by the force of local and federal law enforcement (Krieger 2020). The federal government pushed to keep meat-processing plants open, exposing nonwhite migrant workers to COVID-19 despite rapid spread in these facilities (Swanson and Yaffe-Bellany 2020). The marginality of migrants was further affirmed through their exclusion from CARES Act relief funds, along with the exclusion of their US citizen relatives living in the same household (National Immigration Forum 2020).

The Crisis and Its Solutions

No Exit: COVID-19 in Carceral Institutions

The pandemic has infected and killed people in prisons and detention centers at far higher rates than it has affected the overall population. People in prisons and detention centers have been infected by COVID-19 at more than five times the rate of the overall population. This disparity has not been evenly distributed. Some states have avoided significant outbreaks, while a majority have seen widespread infections and deaths. Fifteen states have infection rates in prison that are at least seven times higher than the rates in the total state population (see fig. 1). As a result of these outbreaks, the pandemic has disproportionately exposed prisoners and detainees to premature death. The death rate in prisons as of October 2020 was 105 per 100,000, compared to 66 per 100,000 in the general population. By January 2021, the overall death rate had skyrocketed to 135 per 100,000, but the death rate in prison had risen to at least 188 per 100,000.[1]

This death rate differential, however, understates the disparity. The pandemic poses the greatest harm to older populations, especially those 65+ years old. But this demographic constitutes a relatively small percentage of the prison population. In June 2020 Brendan Saloner and colleagues adjusted the COVID-19 deaths in prison to account for the age demographics. They estimated how many prison deaths would occur if the death rate in prisons were the same within each age group as in the general population. After adjusting for age and gender, prison deaths were three times higher than in the overall population. We replicated this analysis in October 2020, and the gap had persisted, despite national deaths surpassing 200,000. After adjusting for age, prisoners are more than three times more

---

1. See the online-only appendix for more on data sources. Because the prison population dropped significantly after the pandemic began, the denominator (prison population numbers from earlier in the pandemic) likely deflates the death rate in prisons.

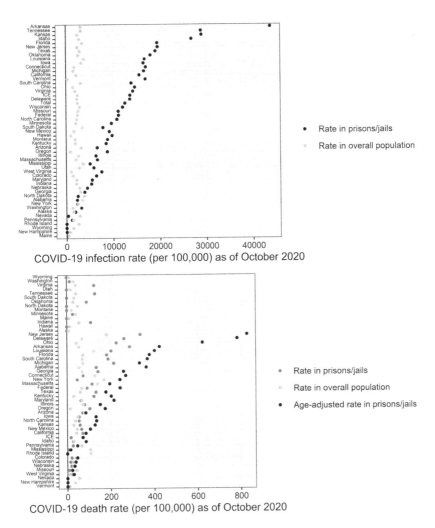

Figure 1 COVID-19 infection rates and death rates by state in prison and overall population as of October 2020.

Sources: Centers for Disease Control, Marshall Project, Census Bureau, state-level reports on incarcerated population.

likely to die from COVID-19. We also collected age distributions of prison populations and COVID-19 death rates by age within each state to conduct this analysis on the state level. We found a similar trend: at least seven states have exposed incarcerated people to rates of death at least five times more than their peers in the state as a whole (see fig. 1). Once outbreaks spread in prisons and detention centers, infections spread at a deadly pace, leaving the disproportionately Black and Latinx people in these facilities facing compounding racial vulnerability.[2]

At the root of the COVID-19 crisis inside carceral institutions lies a combination of policy failures, institutional abandonment, and government malfeasance. A report from the Marshall Project and *Vice News* described conditions inside Federal Correctional Institution at Elkon, Ohio, this way: "The conditions there were ripe for an outbreak, as dozens of men were packed into a dorm with stacked bunk beds, no hot water, and no access to the outdoors or sunlight for weeks." Against CDC recommendations, prison authorities have continually mixed sick and healthy individuals with little physical distance between them (Blakinger and Hamilton 2020). Despite the CDC's call to provide personal protective equipment (PPE), face masks were slow to arrive, and when they did, they were often of poor quality.

Inmate transfers and admissions continued despite the pandemic raging inside. After a series of COVID-19 outbreaks triggered by inmate transfers in March, as was the case with San Quentin, the federal Bureau of Prisons placed a lockdown on new transfers across 122 facilities (Johnson 2020). In May these restrictions were officially lifted with 6,800 new admissions. Even during the active period of the March directive, however, transfers continued seemingly unabated across the country without proper testing or preventive measures (Phillips 2020). Detainee transfers had particularly harsh impacts in immigrant detention facilities. Between March and June, the Marshall Project and the *New York Times* counted more than 750 domestic flights carrying migrants under the custody of Immigration and Customs Enforcement (ICE). Despite the rapid spread rate, reports from both federal and state prisons show a lack of testing taking place behind bars (Kassie and Marcolini 2020; Rubin, Golden, and Webster 2020).

#FreeThemAll: Demands for Decarceration and Harm Reduction

The stories coming out of carceral facilities show both the deplorable conditions that led to COVID-19 clusters but also the centrality of inmate activism in advocating for better conditions. As of February 1, 2021, the University of California, Los Angeles, Law COVID-19 Behind Bars Data

2. See section 1 of the online-only appendix for state-by-state data and more information about these data. The variation across states reveals the differences in how state governments protected inmates with varying levels of effectiveness. Such variation highlights our broader point, since many of the primary actors are at the state and local levels. While this variation across states deserves in-depth treatment, it is beyond the scope of what we can provide here.

Project counts 229 "grassroots and other COVID-19 related efforts" and 75 "correctional population reduction requests" (Dolovich 2020). For its part, the organization Freedom for Immigrants (2020) reports 63 organizing campaigns within migrant detention centers related to COVID-19. The demands embodied by lawsuits, protests, and hunger strikes inside and outside prisons are ideologically diverse — going from reformism to prison abolitionism. An exploration of the various advocacy campaigns mentioned above reveals three main types of policy demands espoused by these campaigns:

First, there is a demand for harm-reduction practices inside carceral institutions. These include the provision of PPE, COVID-19 testing, social distancing, guaranteed services (e.g., commissaries and phone calls), and proper sanitation. The purpose of these policies is to prevent the spread of COVID-19, provide proper care for those with the virus, and procure safe living conditions in the middle of the pandemic. Harm-reduction practices are exemplified in a list of demands put together by the advocacy organization Survived and Punished (2020) to improve conditions inside the California Institution for Women: "Ensure that all incarcerated people, including those in COVID-19 quarantine, have daily access to food, clean water, and non-punitive medical care, including mental health care. . . . Immediately and freely distribute non-diluted cleaning and disinfecting supplies."

Advocacy campaigns have also embraced demands around crisis decarceration. The purpose of these policies is to reduce the total population inside prisons and ameliorate the risk of COVID-19 spread (see Wang et al. 2020). These include calls to release elderly and physically vulnerable patients, including those with respiratory illnesses. Or, as the list of demands by Survived and Punished (2020) put it, "Release all elderly (50+) and medically high-risk people to safe quarantine outside of prison." They also involve policies that expand release eligibility, such as those pushed and eventually implemented in the state of California (Myers and Willon 2020). Crisis decarceration demands also include a halt to new admissions and transfers across and within facilities. Pressed between a rock and a hard place, organizers inside migrant detention centers demanded expedited deportations for detainees with no more appeals or legal recourse (Narea 2020).

Finally, some organizations used the COVID-19 crisis to critique the criminal justice system's legitimacy through abolitionist decarceration demands. Whereas calls for crisis decarceration encompassed short-term policies, abolitionist decarceration demands asked for the release of all prisoners and for the abolition of incarceration as a tool of criminal justice altogether. Describing the effects of COVID-19 in carceral institutions, the Detention Watch Network campaign guidelines read: "Demand Freedom for All! This moment highlights why cages are a public health nuisance, people can't heal, recuperate, or avoid infection in jails and prisons. No one will get release unless we demand everyone be released" (DWN 2020: 2).

Public Views of the Crisis

We identified three phases of compounding racialized vulnerability: racially unequal exposure to death, an external shock that poses greater risk to vulnerable people, and poor responses to this external event that exacerbate harm. We investigate these dynamics in the context of public opinion during the COVID-19 crisis. We find that the general public places less priority on the lives of prisoners and shows reticence toward responses that involve releasing people from carceral institutions. In other words, there is reluctance to support responses that undo the disparities that created racialized vulnerability in the first place, even though there is general support for improving conditions during the crisis. However, information about the preexisting racial disparities increases support for more extensive solutions during the crisis. In this way, our survey offers a modest picture of public support for structural changes, and it also suggests that the pandemic can expose racial vulnerability such that appeals to racial disparities shift views toward more extensive responses.

Data and Methods

We conducted two surveys of American adults fielded in April and May 2020. The surveys were fielded on Lucid, a web-based survey platform. These modules were included as a part of the Yale Cooperative Lucid Surveys. Respondents were recruited through a diverse array of online methods, including digital ads and mobile games. The surveys employed a quota-based sampling method, and this created demographically diverse samples that closely approximate the US population. We also incorporated weights to improve the correspondence of the data to the general population according to age, gender, household income, racial group, region, and education level (see appendix 2.1 in the online-only appendix). We present the weighted findings for our descriptive analysis, and we present our unweighted findings for our experimental analysis. We present alternative analyses in the online-only appendix, in addition to a table with demographic summaries of the survey sample (see tables 4 and 5).

The first survey measured views on COVID-19 in prisons and jails, and the second survey measured views on COVID-19 in immigrant detention centers. The first survey was conducted in April 2020, and 1,040 American adults completed it. In the first survey, all participants were given the following text before answering the questions:

> Many public health experts have identified prisons and jails as sites vulnerable to COVID-19 outbreaks. Steps have been taken to reduce the prison population. While advocates have called for more people to be released, opponents of such measures argue that it is unsafe to release people convicted of crimes as well as unfair to crime victims.

After participants received this information, we asked a series of questions about respondents' views on COVID-19 in prisons and jails. We started with general questions, and then we presented a series of policy proposals to measure support for these proposals. We followed this with some general questions about incarceration in the United States (see appendix 2.2.1 in the online-only appendix for the full list of questions).

The second survey was conducted in May 2020, and 1,080 American adults completed it. In the second survey, all participants were given the following prompt:

> Many public health experts have identified immigrant detention centers as sites vulnerable to COVID-19 outbreaks. Such outbreaks have begun in many immigrant detention centers across the country. At least 47 detention centers have witnessed cases of COVID.

After participants received this information, we asked respondents about their general views of COVID-19 in detention centers, and we followed with questions about policy preferences, concluding with questions related to broader views of immigration enforcement (see appendix 2.2.2 in the online-only appendix for the full list of questions).

Both surveys embedded experiments, so we could infer the causal effects of different types of information. In the treatment condition, the initial prompt was supplemented with additional information. In the first survey, we randomly provided information about racial disparities in prison. In the second survey, we randomly provided information about poor health conditions in immigrant detention centers. In this section, we provide a description of views on COVID-19 in prisons/jails and detention centers based on these surveys. Then we provide an analysis of the causal effects of the informational treatments.

Description of Views

Devaluation of Lives. In light of the risks posed by the pandemic, we investigated how people valued the lives of those in prisons, jails, and migrant detention centers. To do this, we began each survey with a question on general views on COVID-19 in prisons, jails, and immigrant detention centers. In the first survey, we asked participants, "Which of the following best describes what you think about COVID-19 in prisons?" Respondents were given five options: (1) "Since inmates are guilty of crimes, this is a part of the punishment for their crimes," (2) "Prisons should not be a priority at this time," (3) "This is a serious problem, but protecting those outside prison should be prioritized over protecting those in prison," (4) "This is a public health emergency, and the well-being of prisoners should take a high priority," and (5) "Don't know/No opinion." A plurality of respondents (42.5%) said that COVID-19 in prisons is a serious problem, but that protecting those outside prison should take priority. Another 17.1% of respondents said it is not a priority (11.4%) or that it is a part of punishment for crime (5.7%). Less than a third of respondents (30.2%) said that this is a public health emergency and the well-being of prisoners should take a high priority.[3]

The second survey showed similar patterns with reference to immigrant detainees. We asked survey participants, "Which of the following best describes what you think about COVID-19 in immigrant detention centers?" Respondents were given four options: (1) "We should address COVID-19 inside detention centers to protect the human rights of detainees," (2) "We should address COVID-19 inside detention centers to prevent spread to American citizens," (3) "COVID-19 in detention centers should not be our priority because the detainees are not American," and (4) "Immigrants in detention should bear COVID-19 as part of their punishment for coming to the US without authorization." In this survey, around half of respondents (49.5%) said that we ought to address COVID-19 in detention centers because it is a human rights issue. The other half indicated that immigrants in detention should not be a priority or should be a priority to protect American citizens. Thirty-eight percent said that we ought to address COVID-19 in detention centers to prevent spread to American citizens; 7.9% said that immigrant detainees should not be prioritized because they are not citizens; and 4.2% said that COVID-19 is a part of their punishment for coming to the United States without authorization.

3. When presenting summary descriptive measures, we include both the treatment and control groups. As the coefficient plots in figure 5 show, this does not significantly affect our results, except in the case of policy preferences related to decarceration. In this case, including only the control group widens the gap we highlight between support for harm reduction and support for decarceration.

Across these two surveys, one major theme emerged from this question: a majority of people either give less priority or secondary priority to the lives of people in prisons, jails, and detention centers. Most respondents believe either that we ought not prioritize protecting people in these places or that it should be a priority to protect other people whom they may infect. Prisoners are among the most vulnerable to COVID-19; yet, on average, respondents view them as less worthy of care and protection, without the same inherent value as nonprisoners. Public opinion mirrors—and sanctions—the governmental responses described above and reinforces the process of compounding racialized vulnerability: the lives of the already vulnerable behind bars face compounded harm by the lack of priority given to their lives amidst the pandemic.

Policy Preferences on Harm Reduction and Decarceration. After measuring general views, we asked about support for a series of policy proposals roughly mirroring activist demands. These policy proposals included proposals related to harm reduction (increased sanitation, more testing, medical care) and decarceration (releasing already eligible, releasing vulnerable, and releasing as many as possible). Respondents were given the opportunity to say whether they agreed with each proposal on a five-point scale ranging from "Strongly Disagree" to "Strongly Agree." We converted responses to a numeric scale from 0 to 4, with strongly agree equal to 4 and strongly disagree equal to 0. We provide the weighted means in our summary measures, and we provide the unweighted results in the online-only appendix (see figs. 14–15 and 23–24) with similar trends present. We provide the weighted means in our summary measures, and we also combine the proportion that agree and strongly agree to create a dichotomous measure of policy support. We provide the unweighted results in the online-only appendix. Three major themes emerged from these policy responses.

First, there was general support for harm reduction, but much less support for decarceration. The weighted mean support for better sanitation in prisons was 3.11, and mean support for increased testing was 2.9. More precisely, 76% of respondents either strongly favored or favored providing increased sanitation supplies and personal protective equipment in prisons and jails. A slightly smaller majority (61% of respondents) also expressed support for ensuring that people released from prison receive necessary preventative care and medical treatment (see fig. 2).

Similar patterns held true in questions about harm reduction in immigrant detention centers. The weighted mean response for providing increased

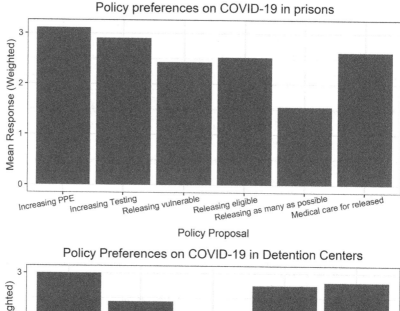

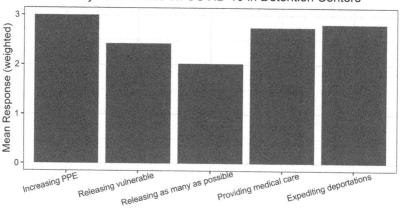

Figure 2 Policy preferences on COVID-19 in prisons and detention centers.

sanitation supplies and personal protective equipment was 3, and the mean response for providing medical care for released people was 2.81. Seventy percent of respondents strongly favored or favored providing increased sanitation supplies and PPE in detention centers, and 62% of respondents favored providing medical care for released people (see fig. 2).

We found much less support for releasing incarcerated people or immigrants in detention. The weighted mean response was 2.43 for releasing those already eligible and 2.53 for releasing vulnerable populations (including elderly people and pregnant women). The weighted mean support for releasing as many as possible was 1.55. In other words, 56% of respondents said they strongly agree or agree with the proposal to release people already eligible for release, and only 25% of respondents agreed or strongly agreed with the proposal to release as many people as possible (see fig. 2).

Detention centers received similar responses. The mean 50% of respondents strongly favored or favored releasing vulnerable populations, and 35% strongly favored or favored releasing as many people as possible. Both surveys confirm strong support for harm reduction but deep reluctance toward releasing people from carceral institutions.

Second, there was a strong correlation between policy preferences and the valuation of the lives of people in prisons and detention centers. As people placed less value and priority on addressing COVID-19 in these institutions, they consistently expressed less support for policies that would promote the well-being of prisoners and detainees (see appendix figs. 16 and 25 in the online-only appendix for regression coefficient plots). The weighted mean support for better sanitation increased from 2.22 to 3.08 when moving from those who said it is a part of the punishment for crimes committed and those who consider prisoners' lives to be a high priority during the crisis. This difference was even more pronounced in preferences related to decarceration. For instance, the mean support for releasing the vulnerable was 1.8 among those who did not consider COVID-19 in prisons a high priority, while it was 2.78 among those who considered it an emergency and priority (see fig. 3).

This is true in connection to immigrant detention centers as well. Among respondents who said COVID-19 in detention centers is a human rights issue, 75% strongly agreed with increasing sanitation supplies and personal protective equipment. For everyone else, only 35% of respondents strongly agreed with this proposal (see fig. 3). These differences were starker for questions related to release. Respondents who indicate that people in prisons and detention centers should not be as prioritized as others are far more likely to say people should not be released. Only one policy preference did not show a correlation across general views of COVID-19 in migrant detention centers: expediting deportations (see appendix fig. 25 in the online-only appendix). We believe this unlikely convergence of preferences to be the result of divergent beliefs. On the one hand, respondents who prioritize the health of migrant detainees may be heeding the political

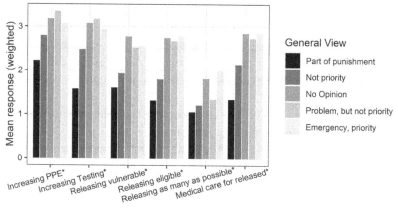

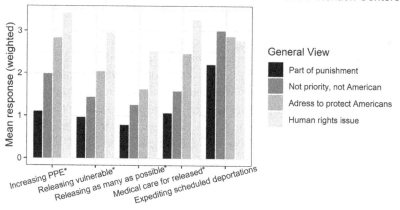

Figure 3 Policy preferences conditioned on general views of COVID-19 in prisons and detention centers.

Note: * indicates statistically significant correlation (p < .05) between general view and policy preference.

demands of migrant detainees and advocates.[4] Respondents regarding the health of migrant detainees as a low priority may favor deportations out of a nativist preference for a higher net rate of deportations.

4. Detainees in Bristol County, Massachusetts, for example, demanded expedited deportation for consenting migrants who had no further legal recourse as part of their protest efforts (Narea 2020).

Overall, these findings show the correlation between the priority given to the lives of people in carceral institutions and how people believe we ought to respond to this crisis. This corresponds to the work that shows a correlation between racial resentment and opposition to voting rights for people convicted of a felony (Wilson, Owens, and Davis 2011).

Third, white respondents were more likely than Black and Latinx respondents to support harm reduction measures, but Black and Latinx respondents were more likely to support releasing more people from prisons and immigrant detention centers. White respondents were more in favor of increasing sanitation supplies and PPE, but Black and Latinx respondents were much more supportive of proposals to release incarcerated people and slightly more supportive of releasing more detained immigrants (see table 1 and appendix fig. 20).[5] Black-white differences in beliefs about policing and incarceration are well documented (Jefferson, Neuner, and Pasek 2020; Unnever 2008). We extend that work here to cover differences in beliefs regarding releasing people from prisons and jails during the COVID-19 pandemic.

The Effects of Information about Racial Disparities and Health Conditions

We also studied how public views of COVID-19 in prisons and jails were affected by informational treatments. To do this, we randomly assigned half of respondents in each survey to receive a short statement related to prisons/jails or immigrant detention centers. For the first survey, we examined the effect of information about racial disparities in prisons and jails. For the second survey, we examined the effect of information about poor health conditions in migrant detention centers.

Racial Disparities in Prisons and Jails. In the survey module on COVID-19 in prisons and jails, we added the following information to the survey prompt:

Black Americans are incarcerated in the US at a rate that is about 5 times that of White Americans. Thus, it is likely a far greater proportion of the Black population will die in prisons from COVID-19 than the proportion of the White population who will die because of COVID-19 in prisons.

---

5. This graph format featuring the scatterplot and subgroup means is adapted from Coppock 2019.

Table 1   Policy Preferences Related to Sanitation in Prisons and Decarceration during COVID-19 Crisis

	Mean	Strongly disagree	Disagree	Neither agree nor disagree	Agree	Strongly Agree
Increased sanitation in prisons and jails						
Black	2.75	4.8%	12.4%	20%	28.6%	34.3%
Latinx	2.59	5.8%	12.5%	25%	30%	26.7%
Asian	3.00	1.9%	1.9%	16.67%	53.7%	25.9%
White	3.14	2.2%	3%	15.2%	37.7%	41.9%
Other	2.97	3.1%	6.3%	18.8%	34.4%	37.5%
Releasing as many people as possible from prisons and jails						
Black	1.94	17.5%	19%	28.6%	25.7%	9.5%
Latinx	1.74	24.2%	16.7%	30.9%	17.5%	10.8%
Asian	1.98	20.4%	11.1%	33.3%	20.4%	14.8%
White	1.45	31.2%	25.7%	19.7%	13.7%	9.7%
Other	1.66	28.1%	18.7%	31.3%	3.1%	18.7%

Notes: Policy preferences related to sanitation and PPE in prisons and jails and decarceration during the COVID-19 crisis. Means are measured by converting responses to a 5-point scale from strongly disagree (0) to strongly agree (4).

This information communicated the first phase of compounding racialized vulnerabilities: preexisting racial disparities in outcomes. We analyzed the differences in views related to COVID-19 in prisons and jails between those in the control group and those who received this prompt. We conducted ordinary least squares (OLS) regressions, and we included a variety of pretreatment covariates as control variables (see appendix tables 6–15 in the online-only appendix for full regression tables).

In questions related to harm reduction, this information about racial disparities had no significant effect. But people who received the informational treatment were more likely to favor releasing more people. The treatment increased agreement with releasing the vulnerable by 0.11 on a five-point scale (though this was not significant). It significantly increased agreement with releasing those already eligible by 0.21, and it significantly increased agreement with releasing as many people as possible by 0.23 (see fig. 4).

These causal effects are large and important. In the control group, 58% of respondents disagreed or strongly disagreed with the proposal to release

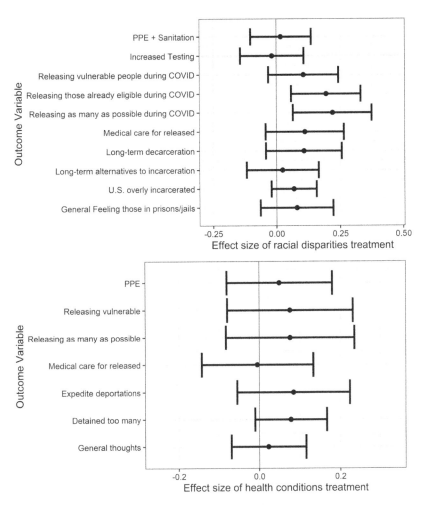

Figure 4 Coefficient plots for effects of informational treatments on views of COVID-19 in prisons and detention centers.

as many people as possible. In the treatment group, this fell to 48%. The effect size for releasing the eligible is equivalent to a shift of three points on a seven-point party ID scale, and the effect size for releasing as many people as possible is equivalent to a four-point shift in party ID (e.g., from a weak Republican to a weak Democrat).[6] These effects partially

6. See appendix table 8, model 6, in the online-only appendix. The Lin estimator normalizes coefficients and allows for this kind of comparison.

closed the gap between support for harm reduction and support for decarceration during COVID-19.

This effect was concentrated among white and Latinx respondents (see fig. 5).[7] In the control group, Black respondents were far more likely than white respondents to support releasing people from prisons and jails, and Latinx respondents were between the Black and white respondents. But the racial disparities treatment dramatically changed these differences. The treatment had a large and significant positive effect on white and Latinx respondents, increasing their support for releasing people from prisons and jails. But it had the opposite effect on Black respondents, who were less likely to support releasing people from prison as a result of the treatment (though this effect was insignificant).

Previous research has found that information about racial disparities in the criminal justice system does not change views on the criminal justice system (Hetey and Eberhardt 2018). Respondents can simply fit information about racial disparities within their views of the world. For instance, racial disparities can fit within conceptions of Black criminality and the dehumanization of Black people (Jardina and Piston 2019; Unnever and Cullen 2010). For others, these disparities reinforce existing opposition to systemic racism within the criminal justice system (Hetey and Eberhardt 2018). But in the context of COVID-19, information about racial disparities—with no additional commentary as to why these disparities exist—changed views. It would make sense that Black Americans' views do not change with this informational treatment because they are already aware of these disparities. For others, this stark disparity combines with the death resulting from COVID-19 to prompt reconsideration of our continued patterns of incarceration.

Poor Health Conditions and Immigrant Detention Centers. In the survey module about COVID-19 in immigrant detention centers, we randomly assigned half of respondents to receive this prompt:

Conditions inside immigration detention centers do not allow for social distancing or proper hygiene. Large groups of people are often placed in one room with 3 ft. between beds. Common complaints include lack of

---

7. In figure 6, we show heterogenous effects by respondent racial group. We include Black, white, and Latinx respondent groups in this analysis. Our small sample sizes are relatively small in other groups, and this limits the statistical power needed to include these other groups in this analysis.

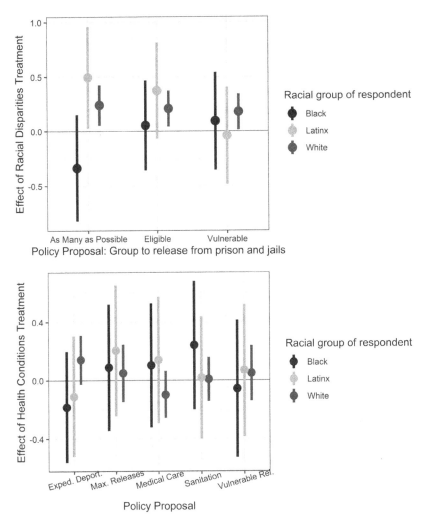

Figure 5 Coefficient plots of treatment effects by racial group.

soap, malfunctioning bathrooms, and improper medical care. Researchers suggest that without proper measures, 70 percent of ICE detainees may become infected over a 90-day period.

We hypothesized that this information could prompt people to increase support for harm reduction, given the poor conditions that currently exist. We also hypothesized that this could increase support for releasing immigrants from detention, since it could be seen as a way to save lives.

However, this information did not have a significant effect on views of COVID-19 in immigrant detention centers (see fig. 4).[8] For questions relating to increasing PPE, releasing as many as possible, medical care for the released, and general thoughts on COVID-19 in immigrant detention centers, the estimate of the effect was less than 0.03 from 0 and not significant. The estimates were slightly larger for questions related to releasing the vulnerable ($t = 0.049$), expediting deportations ($t = 0.085$), and whether the United States has detained too many people ($t = 0.07$). The treatment effects are consistently positive across all but one of the outcome variables, but these estimates are fairly small and statistically insignificant. They are suggestive that the treatment may shift preferences, but any shift would be small. And the lack of significance prevents us from making any conclusive claims about the positive effects. (See fig. 5 for heterogeneous effects by respondent racial group.)

Conclusion

We have sketched a picture of the politics surrounding COVID-19 inside carceral institutions through the lens of compounding racial vulnerability. The roots of the crisis predate the virus; mass incarceration and structural racism are the underlying conditions that have rendered nonwhite detainees "vulnerable to premature death" (Gilmore 2007: 28). Institutional responses at multiple levels have heightened structural marginalization to bring about new forms of compounding racial vulnerability, often sanctioned by an electorate unwilling to protect the health of inmates and detainees. However, we also hope to amplify the vigorous organizing happening inside and outside these institutions, centering decarceration demands that have become even more prominent in the aftermath of the marches that followed the killing of George Floyd. Our survey results illustrate compounding racial vulnerability by showing the low priority given to conditions inside prisons and detention centers compared to other aspects of public life during the pandemic. We also show widespread approval for harm-reduction measures but more opposition to decarceration. Our work shows that messages highlighting racial disparities may have an effect on public support for prisoner release. It is our hope that rather than seeing these findings as a display of static opposition or infeasibility of activist demands, advocates and academics alike may see our work as a springboard to inform campaigns around carceral and racial justice.

---

8. See appendix tables 16–22 in the online-only appendix for full regression tables.

▪ ▪ ▪

Matthew G. T. Denney is a PhD candidate in political science at Yale University. He studies race, policing, and faith in politics and communities. matthew.denney@yale.edu.

Ramon Garibaldo Valdez is a PhD candidate at Yale University researching immigrant organizing, social movements, and racial authoritarianism. ramon.garibaldo@yale.edu

Acknowledgments

We would like to thank Ray Block Jr. for tremendous support through various stages of this project. We also want to thank others who provided helpful feedback and support: Danny Hirschel-Burns, Dasean Nardone-White, Gwen Prowse, panel participants at the 2020 APSA meeting, editors, anonymous reviewers, Alex Coppock, Kyle Peyton, Roselyn Cruz, and Lara Takasugi Denney. Lastly, we would like to acknowledge the organizers in prisons and detention centers who have inspired this work.

References

Adamy, Janet. 2020. "Coronavirus, Economic Toll Threaten to Worsen Black Mortality Rates." *Wall Street Journal*, June 13. www.wsj.com/articles/coronavirus-economic-toll-threaten-to-worsen-black-mortality-rates-11592046000.

Alexander, Michelle. 2010. *The New Jim Crow: Mass Incarceration in an Age of Colorblindness*. New York: New Press.

APM Research Lab. 2020. "The Color of Coronavirus: COVID-19 Deaths by Race and Ethnicity in the US." September 16. www.apmresearchlab.org/covid/deaths-by-race.

Bailey, Zinzi D., Nancy Krieger, Madina Agenor, Jasmine Graces, Natalia Linos, and Mary T. Bassett. 2017. "Structural Racism and Health Inequities in the USA: Evidence and Interventions." *Lancet* 389, no. 10077: 1453–63.

Blakinger, Keri, and Keegan Hamilton. 2020. "'I Begged Them to Let Me Die': How Federal Prisons Became Coronavirus Death Traps." Marshall Project, June 18. www.themarshallproject.org/2020/06/18/i-begged-them-to-let-me-die-how-federal-prisons-became-coronavirus-death-traps.

BondGraham, Darwin. 2007. "The New Orleans that Race Built: Racism, Disaster, and Urban Spatial Relationships." *Souls: A Critical Journal of Black Politics, Culture, and Society* 9, no. 1: 4–18.

Bonilla-Silva, Eduardo. 1997. "Rethinking Racism: Toward a Structural Interpretation." *American Sociological Review* 62, no. 3: 465–80.

CDC (Centers for Disease Control and Prevention). 2021. "COVID Data Tracker." covid.cdc.gov/covid-data-tracker/#vaccination-demographic (accessed February 26, 2021).

Clayton, Abene. 2020. "San Quentin Faces California's Deadliest Prison Outbreak after Latest COVID Fatalities." *Guardian*, August 4. www.theguardian.com/us-news /2020/aug/04/san-quentin-covid-19-deaths-prison-outbreak.

Coppock, Alexander. 2019. "Visualize as You Randomize: Design-Based Statistical Graphs for Randomized Experiments." In *Advances in Experimental Political Science*, edited by James N. Druckman and Donald P. Green, 320–38. Cambridge: Cambridge University Press.

Dickerson, Caitlin. 2020. "Vulnerable Border Community Battles Virus on 'A Straight Up Trajectory.'" *New York Times*, July 19 (updated July 22). www.nytimes.com /2020/07/19/us/coronavirus-texas-rio-grande-valley.html?smid=em-share.

Dolovich, Sharon. 2020. "UCLA Law Covid-19 Behind Bars Data Project." docs .google.com/spreadsheets/d/1X6uJkXXS-O6eePLxw2e4JeRtM41uPZ2eRcOA_ HkPVTk/edit?fbclid=IwAR2EgtwoAI_cRoPnibu77YH9Fl-fDoJVk9mh1Dwkx 048ln_tgqC_2dSht0w#gid=1720501154 (accessed April 22, 2021).

Du Bois, W. E. B. (1903) 2003. *The Souls of Black Folk*. Penn State Electronic Classic Series, 2016. www.yumpu.com/en/document/view/47176817/the-souls-of-black -folk-dr-earl-wright-ii.

DWN (Detention Watch Network). 2020. "#FreeThemAll: Toolkit to Support Local Demands for Mass Release of People in ICE Custody." docs.google.com/document /d/1d5O71qvC3-xkwGO3F61cLytjoVgzBohs18RP2LvV6LM/edit (accessed May 20, 2021).

Figueroa, Jose F., Rishi K. Wadhera, Dennis Lee, Robert W. Yeh, and Benjamin D. Sommers. 2020. "Community-Level Factors Associated with Racial and Ethnic Disparities in COVID-19 Rates in Massachusetts." *Health Affairs* 39, no. 11. doi.org/ 10.1377/hlthaff.2020.01040.

Freedom for Immigrants. 2020. "Mapping US Immigration Detention." www.free domforimmigrants.org/map (accessed April 22, 2021).

Frymer, Paul, Dara Z. Strolovitch, and Dorian T. Warren. 2006. "New Orleans Is Not the Exception: Re-Politicizing the Study of Racial Inequality." *DuBois Review* 3, no. 1: 37–57.

Gilmore, Ruth Wilson. 2007. *Golden Gulag: Prison, Surplus, Crisis, and Opposition in Globalizing California*. Berkeley: University of California Press.

Golash-Boza, Tanya M. 2015. *Deported: Immigrant Policing, Disposable Labor, and Global Capitalism*. New York: New York University Press.

Gottschalk, Marie. 2015. *Caught: The Prison State and the Lockdown of American Politics*. Princeton, NJ: Princeton University Press.

Hadden, Sally. 2003. *Slave Patrols: Law and Violence in Virginia and the Carolinas*. Cambridge, MA: Harvard University Press.

Hetey, Rebecca C., and Jennifer L. Eberhardt. 2018. "The Numbers Don't Speak for Themselves: Racial Disparities and the Persistence of Inequality in the Criminal Justice System." *Current Directions in Psychological Science* 27, no. 3: 183–87. doi.org/10.1177/0963721418763931.

Jardina, Ashley, and Spencer Piston. 2019. "The Dehumanization of Blacks and White Support for Punitive Criminal Justice Policy." Paper presented at the "American Politics and Public Policy Workshop," Institution for Social and Policy Studies, New Haven, CT, November 6.

Jefferson, Hakeem, Fabian G. Neuner, and Josh Pasek. 2020. "Seeing Blue in Black and White: Race and Perceptions of Officer-Involved Shootings." *Perspectives on Politics*, December 4. doi.org/10.1017/S1537592720003618.

Johnson, Kevin. 2020. "Federal Prison Officers Order System-Wide Lockdown in Bid to Limit Coronavirus Spread." *USA Today*, March 31. www.usatoday.com/story /news/politics/2020/03/31/coronavirus-federal-prison-officials-order-system-wide -lockdown/5100375002/.

Kassie, Emily, and Barbara Marcolini. 2020. "How ICE Exported the Coronavirus." Marshall Project, July 10. www.themarshallproject.org/2020/07/10/how-ice-exported -the-coronavirus.

Krieger, Nancy. 2020. "ENOUGH: COVID-19, Structural Racism, Police Brutality, Plutocracy, Climate Change—and Time for Health Justice, Democratic Governance, and an Equitable, Sustainable Future." *American Journal of Public Health* 110, no. 11: 949–51.

Lerman, Amy E., and Vesla M. Weaver. 2014. *Arresting Citizenship: The Democratic Consequences of American Crime Control*. Chicago: University of Chicago Press.

Lopez, William D. 2019. *Separated: Family and Community in the Aftermath of an Immigration Raid*. Baltimore, MD: Johns Hopkins University Press.

Macias-Rojas, Patrisia. 2016. *From Deportation to Prison: The Politics of Immigration Enforcement in Post–Civil Rights America*. New York: New York University Press.

Marshall Project. 2020. "A State-by-State Look at Coronavirus in Prisons." October 29. www.themarshallproject.org/2020/05/01/a-state-by-state-look-at-coronavirus -in-prisons.

Moreno Haines, Juan. 2020. "At San Quentin, a Desperate Man Goes on Hunger Strike to Protest Conditions in a COVID-19 Isolation Unit." Solitary Watch, August 10. solitarywatch.org/2020/08/10/at-san-quentin-a-desperate-man-goes-on-hunger-strike -to-protest-conditions-in-a-covid-19-isolation-unit/.

Moreno Haines, Juan, and Elizabeth Weill-Greenberg. 2020. "At San Quentin, Overcrowding Laid the Groundwork for an Explosive COVID-19 Outbreak." *Appeal*, July 21. theappeal.org/at-san-quentin-overcrowding-laid-the-groundwork-for-an -explosive-covid-19-outbreak/.

Myers, John, and Phil Willon. 2020. "California to Release 8,000 prisoners in Hopes of Easing Coronavirus Crisis." *Los Angeles Times*, July 10. www.latimes.com /california/story/2020-07-10/california-release-8000-prisoners-coronavirus-crisis -newsom.

Narea, Nicole. 2020. "Immigrant Detainees in Massachusetts Are Fighting to Be Released in the Pandemic." *Vox*, April 9. www.vox.com/2020/4/9/21207346/corona virus-immigrant-ice-detention-massachusetts-bristol.

National Immigration Forum. 2020. "Fact Sheet: Mixed Status Families and COVID-19 Economic Relief." August 12. immigrationforum.org/article/mixed-status-families -and-covid-19-economic-relief/.

New York Times. 2020. "Coronavirus in the US: Latest Map and Case Count." August 17. www.nytimes.com/interactive/2020/us/coronavirus-us-cases.html#clusters.

Omi, Michael, and Howard Winant. 2015. *Racial Formation in the United States*. 3rd ed. New York: Routledge.

Oppel, Richard, Jr., Robert Gebeloff, K. K. Rebecca Lai, Will Wright, and Mitch Smith. 2020. "The Fullest Look Yet at the Racial Inequality of Coronavirus." *New York Times*, July 5. www.nytimes.com/interactive/2020/07/05/us/coronavirus -latinos-african-americans-cdc-data.html.

Phillips, Kristine. 2020. "Bureau of Prisons to Start Moving 6,800 New Federal Inmates to Its Facilities." *USA Today*, May 22. www.usatoday.com/story/news /politics/2020/05/22/coronavirus-bureau-prisons-move-6–800-new-inmates-its -facilities/5246915002/.

Pirtle, Whitney N. Laster. 2020. "Racial Capitalism: A Fundamental Cause of Novel Coronavirus (COVID-19) Pandemic Inequities in the United States." *Health Education and Behavior* 47, no. 4: 504–8.

Rubin, Anat, Tim Golden, and Richard Webster. 2020. "Inside the US's Largest Maximum Security Prison." ProPublica, June 24. www.propublica.org/article/inside -the-uss-largest-maximum-security-prison-covid-19-raged.

Saloner, Brendan, Kalind Parish, Julie A. Ward, Grace DiLaura, and Sharon Dolovich. 2020. "COVID-19 Cases and Deaths in Federal and State Prisons." *JAMA* 324, no. 6: 602–3. doi.org/10.1001/jama.2020.12528.

Sampaio, Anna. 2015. *Terrorizing Latina/o Immigrants: Race, Gender, and Immigration Politics in the Age of Security*. Philadelphia, PA: Temple University Press.

Sewell, Alyasah Ali. 2020. "Policing the Block: Pandemics, Systemic Racism, and the Blood of America." *City and Community* 19, no. 3: 496–505.

Soss, Joe, and Vesla Weaver. 2017. "Police Are Our Government: Politics, Political Science, and the Policing of Race-Class Subjugated Communities." *Annual Review of Political Science* 20: 565–91.

Stivers, Camilla. 2007. "'So Poor and So Black': Hurricane Katrina, Public Administration, and the Issue of Race." *Public Administration Review* 67, no. 1: 48–56.

Survived and Punished. 2020. "Take Action! California Women's Prison Denying Basic Needs to People in COVID-19 Quarantine." May 19. survivedandpunished .org/event/take-action-california-prison-denying-water-to-incarcerated-people -who-are-covid-19/.

Swanson, Ana, and David Yaffe-Bellany. 2020. "Trump Declares Meat Supply 'Critical,' Aiming to Reopen Plants." *New York Times*, April 28. www.nytimes.com /2020/04/28/business/economy/coronavirus-trump-meat-food-supply.html.

Unnever, James D. 2008. "Two Worlds Far Apart: Black-White Differences in Beliefs about Why African-American Men Are Disproportionately Imprisoned." *Criminology* 46, no. 2: 511–38. doi.org/10.1111/j.1745-9125.2008.00117.x.

Unnever, James D., and Francis T. Cullen. 2010. "The Social Sources of Americans' Punitiveness: A Test of Three Competing Models." *Criminology* 48, no. 1: 99–129. doi.org/10.1111/j.1745-9125.2010.00181.x.

Walker, Mark. 2020. "Pandemic Highlights Deep-Rooted Problems in Indian Health Service." *New York Times*, September 29. www.nytimes.com/2020/09/29/us/politics /coronavirus-indian-health-service.html.

Wang, Emily, Bruce Western, Emily Backes, and Julie Schuck, eds. 2020. *Decarcerating Correctional Facilities during COVID-19: Advancing Health, Equity, and Safety*. Washington, DC: National Academies Press.

Western, Bruce. 2006. *Punishment and Inequality in America*. New York: Russell Sage Foundation.

Williams, Timothy, Libby Seline, and Rebecca Griesbach. 2020. "Coronavirus Cases Rise Sharply in Prisons Even as They Plateau Nationwide." *New York Times*, June 30. www.nytimes.com/2020/06/16/us/coronavirus-inmates-prisons-jails.html.

Wilson, David C., Michael Leo Owens, and Darren Davis. 2011. *Racial Resentment and the Restoration of Voting Rights for Felons*. doi.org/10.2139/ssrn.1904089.

Americans' View of the Impact of COVID-19: Perspectives on Racial Impacts and Equity

Katherine Carman
Anita Chandra
RAND Corporation

Carolyn Miller
Robert Wood Johnson Foundation

Christopher Nelson
Jhacova Williams
RAND Corporation

Abstract

Context: The COVID-19 pandemic has had a disparate effect on African Americans and Latinos. But it is unknown how aware the public is of these differences and how the pandemic has changed perceptions of equity and access to health care.

Methods: We use panel data from nationally representative surveys fielded to the same respondents in 2018 and 2020 to assess views and changes in views over time.

Findings: We found that awareness of inequity is highest among Non-Hispanic Black respondents and higher-income and higher-educated groups, and there have been only small changes in perceptions of inequity over time. However, there have been significant changes in views of the government's obligation to ensure access to health care.

Conclusions: Even in the face of a deadly pandemic, one that has killed disproportionately more African Americans and Latinos, many in the United States continue not to recognize that there are inequities in access to health care and the impact of COVID-19 on certain groups. But policies to address inequity may be shifting. We will continue to follow these respondents to see whether changes in attitudes endure over time or dissipate.

Keywords COVID-19, race, equity, public opinion

The impact of COVID-19 has disproportionately fallen on African American and Hispanic groups, with these groups experiencing higher infection rates, mortality, and financial impacts. Case rates among African Americans are 1.4 times the rates among white Americans, and rates among Hispanic Americans are 1.7 times the rates among white Americans (CDC 2020). This stands on top of long-standing health inequities in the United States. In 2019, for instance, 18.7% of Hispanic Americans and 10.1% of

Journal of Health Politics, Policy and Law, Vol. 46, No. 5, October 2021
DOI 10.1215/03616878-9156033   © 2021 by Duke University Press

African Americans lacked health care access and coverage, compared to 6.3% of whites; and 21% of Hispanic Americans and 17% of African Americans did not see a doctor because of cost in in the past 12 months, compared with 13% of whites (Artiga and Orgera 2019; US Census Bureau 2019). Similar patterns hold for other areas of well-being, such as incarceration and income (Nellis 2016; Wilson 2020).

While inequity in health is well-known and documented in the health fields (IOM 2003), historically it has been less understood by the general public. However, that may be changing. Compared to two years ago, evidence of widespread inequities (in health, education, justice, housing) is now regularly discussed in the mainstream media and in the context of COVID-19; and protests surrounding systemic racism and the deaths of George Floyd, Breonna Taylor, and others have brought increased attention to these disparities. But whether the public appreciates that there are inequities in access to health care related to race, ethnicity, or income, and whether their views have changed as a result of the pandemic, is an open question. This article seeks to assess views of the differential impact of COVID-19, equity in access to health care, and the government's role in addressing access to health care, and how these views may differ across demographic groups and over time.

Braveman and colleagues (2017: 2) state, "Health equity means that everyone has a fair and just opportunity to be as healthy as possible. This requires removing obstacles to health such as poverty, discrimination, and their consequences, including powerlessness and lack of access to good jobs with fair pay, quality education and housing, safe environments, and health care." The public's views and understanding of inequity are key inputs into public policy. Previous studies have shown that political views and perceived costs can be barriers to achieving future policy changes related to equity in health care (Pacheco and Maltby 2017; Pagel et al. 2017).

Increasing polarization in the United States has underscored the ways in which different segments of the population view the same set of conditions and circumstances through different lenses. For instance, a Pew poll found that support for the Black Lives Matter movement remained virtually unchanged among Black Americans between June and September 2021 but fell markedly among white Americans and (to a somewhat lesser extent) among Hispanics (Thomas and Horowitz 2020). Thus it is reasonable to suspect that views of health inequity may differ across racial and other demographic groups. Previous research identifies several factors that influence whether inequity is perceived as a problem and support for government's role in addressing inequity. First, whites often have less diverse networks, providing fewer situational cues about health inequity, a pattern exacerbated by segregation in neighborhoods, schools, and work-places (Kraus, Rucker, and Richeson 2017; Shedd 2015). Second, social structures (e.g., framing of history) leaves Americans motivated to perceive society as fair and just, and this tendency may be stronger for whites, who are often more highly invested in existing social and economic structures (Salter, Adams, and Perez 2018). Motivated cognition related to a colorblind worldview may lead white Americans to underestimate the degree of inequity (Kraus, Rucker, and Richeson 2017; Kraus and Tan 2015; Richeson and Nussbaum 2004).

There is evidence of increasing support for the idea that health care coverage is a government responsibility, with an increase from 51% in 2016 to 60% in 2018. However, deeply rooted cultural narratives about free choice and personal responsibility remain barriers to widespread appreciation for health inequities (Gollust and Lynch 2011; Hook and Markus 2020). One critical challenge is that this value is inconsistent with another value that commonly underlies Americans' beliefs about social policy issues—individualism (Conover and Feldman 1984; Markus 2001). Economic individualism, for example, asserts that success stems from hard work and self-reliance. This core value of personal responsibility, when extended to conceptualizations of health, lends itself to the conclusion that individuals, rather than the government, should be responsible for ensuring their own health (Gollust and Cappella 2014).

Partisan identities can affect the degree to which individuals are willing to support political values such as equal opportunity and self-reliance (Goren, Federico, and Kittilson 2009), which have implications for views about policies to promote health. In addition, political views influence the relative interest in social investment (Citrin 1979). However, the public's willingness to accept these interventions depends on the costs they perceive for themselves, in particular whether they will have to change their own behavior (Diepeveen et al. 2013). Current events also may shift public opinion and attitudes (Krosnick and Kinder 1990). Race, ethnicity, and age are related to the degree to which individuals change their views, with people of color and younger individuals more likely to change their views as a result of media attention (Perrin 2020).

Finally, public opinion can ultimately influence public policy (Burstein 2003). Achieving future policy changes can be supported by a better understanding of the relationship between people's views of inequity and their attitudes about access to health care. According to Ann Swidler (1986: 273), "values remain the major link between culture and action." Thus, if research can help us understand the extent to which the current pandemic has brought a broader awareness and salience of the social determinants of health, including inequity in access to health care, this awareness may create the demand for healthy communities and policies that support them (Jacobs 1992). Ultimately, we would expect these policies to improve overall health and well-being (Aknin et al. 2013; Hessami 2010; Oishi, Schimmack, and Diener 2011).

Using unique panel data, this article contributes to the literature related to COVID-19 by examining how perceptions related to inequity in health care change in the context of the pandemic. These data are ideal for three reasons. First, our data contain responses from the same respondents in two periods—2018 and 2020—allowing us to examine whether respondents change their responses to specific questions asked in both periods (e.g., have their views changed). Second, respondents are asked whether access to health care differed for African Americans and Latinos compared to white Americans in both periods. Examining responses to this question helps us understand how perceptions of inequity in health care differ across demographics and the extent to which perceptions change across periods. We expect people of color experiencing higher inequities in health care to be more likely to report them. Third, surveys in 2020 were fielded in June and July—one month following public outcry and protests over the deaths of George Floyd and Breonna Taylor. These field dates are critical to our understanding of how public perception related to racial inequity can change. Considering that much media attention was devoted to highlighting racial inequity in America following Floyd and Taylor's deaths, we hypothesize that perceptions related to racial inequity are likely to have changed, as the events of 2020 brought increased attention to these inequities.

Using these data, we seek to answer three questions. First, do people perceive racial inequities in health access? Second, is there support for policies that may address racial inequity? And third, do views change over time? For each question, we also address which groups are more or less likely to hold these views. We are particularly interested in understanding groups whose views did not change in light of the pandemic and increased attention to racial inequity.

Methods

Study Design and Sample

Our research draws on longitudinal survey data collected as part of the RAND-RWJF National Survey of Health Attitudes (NSHA) (fielded in 2018) and on the new COVID-19 and the Experiences of Populations at Greater Risk Survey (CEPGRS) (fielded in 2020). While the data used in this article were collected in two separate surveys, the sample for the CEPGRS was drawn from the NSHA.

The NSHA was developed to provide insight into and perspective on how people in the United States think about, value, and prioritize health and consider issues of health equity. These surveys were designed to support measurement of the mindset and expectations of the American public as part of the Robert Wood Johnson Foundation's efforts to measure progress toward achieving a "Culture of Health" (Chandra et al. 2016). Additional information about the NSHA is available in studies by Katherine Grace Carman and others (2016, 2019).

In 2020, as it became clear that COVID-19 and the resulting recession were disproportionately impacting populations historically at greater risk, including people of color and lower-income households, the CEPGRS was developed to provide greater insight into the impact of the pandemic on vulnerable households and on the views of the general public as they relate to health, equity, and the impacts of COVID-19. Several key survey questions from the NSHA were included in the CEPGRS, allowing for longitudinal analysis. Additional information about the CEPGRS is available in Carman et al. 2020.

Both the NSHA and CEPGRS were fielded to the RAND American Life Panel (ALP), a nationally representative internet panel recruited via probability-based sampling methods (see Pollard and Baird 2017 for additional information).[1] To ensure representativeness, computers and internet connections are provided for respondents who do not already have them. Respondents are compensated for completing surveys, receiving $10 for a 15-minute survey, prorated for shorter or longer surveys.

Respondents to the CEPGRS were selected from the NSHA, with an oversample of lower- and middle-income, Black, and Hispanic respondents.[2] The CEPGRS had two versions, with those from populations historically at greater risk receiving more questions about the impact of the COVID-19 pandemic on their personal situation, and others receiving primarily questions about their views. Table 1 summarizes key details of each survey.

We merged the two surveys together and calculated weights to align the characteristics of our sample in 2020 to the 2019 Current Population Survey (CPS) and to account for attrition between the two waves. Our weighting procedure is the same procedure used for other ALP surveys

---

1. Both surveys were also fielded on the KnowledgePanel; however, we are not able to follow respondents over time in the KnowledgePanel. As such, we have focused this article on the American Life Panel.

2. The sample for the 2018 NSHA included respondents from the 2015 NSHA; as a result, neither survey (NSHA or CEPGRS) includes respondents who were 18 or younger in 2015 (born in 1997 or later).

Table 1 Description of Surveys

	NSHA	CEPGRS
Field dates	July 11 to August 30, 2018	June 29 to July 22, 2020
Number of questions*	34	30 or 37
Average survey length	19 minutes	9 or 13 minutes
Number invited	2,858	2,308
Number responded	2,479	1,854
Participation rate	86.7%	80.3%

* Many questions include tables with multiple subquestions or subparts.

and is described in more detail (Pollard and Baird 2017). We aimed to match population proportions on interactions of gender and race and ethnicity, gender and education, and gender and age as well as household income interacted with household size. Appendix table 1 in the online appendix provides results from a regression predicting retention in the sample as a function of demographic characteristics; with the exception of age, which we adjust for in our weighting procedure, we find that demographic characteristics do not predict retention.

Nomenclature

In this article we discuss historically underserved groups in two different contexts: as survey respondents and as groups specifically indicated in our survey questions. When referring to respondent groups, we will include the word *respondents*, and when referring to historically underserved groups that are mentioned in survey questions, we will refer to *indicated groups*. Some analysis will simultaneously refer to similar racial or ethnic groups as both respondents and as the indicated group. When discussing respondents, we will refer to non-Hispanic Black and Hispanic (which is how we define our racial and ethnic groups to create mutually exclusive groups), but when discussing indicated groups, we will refer to African Americans and Latinos. The latter language matches that used in our survey questions and is used because it is clearer for survey participants.

Survey Instrument

Our surveys asked a number of questions about how race and ethnicity impact health, particularly in light of the pandemic. The full text of the 2018 and 2020 surveys are available in studies by Carman and colleagues (2019 and 2020, respectively).

In 2020 respondents were asked about whether they agreed or disagreed (on a five-point Likert scale with 1 representing strongly agree and 5 representing strongly disagree) that the pandemic had a greater impact on people of color.

> People of color (e.g., African Americans, Latinos) are facing more of the health impact of coronavirus (COVID-19) than whites.
>
> People of color (e.g., African Americans, Latinos) are facing more of the financial impact of coronavirus (COVID-19) than whites.

In 2018 and 2020, we asked respondents four questions about their views of equity of access to health care for different demographic groups. These questions were developed for the NSHA in conjunction with NORC at the University of Chicago and have been used in the NSHA as well as the American Health Values Survey (Bye, Ghiradelli, and Fontes 2016).

> When African Americans need health care, do you think it is easier or harder for them to get the care they need than it is for White Americans, or is there not much of a difference?
>
> When Latinos need health care, do you think it is easier or harder for them to get the care they need than it is for White Americans, or is there not much of a difference?
>
> When low-income Americans need health care, do you think it is easier or harder for them to get the care they need than it is for those who are better off financially, or is there not much of a difference?
>
> When Americans living in rural communities need health care, do you think it is easier or harder for them to get the care they need than it is for those who live in urban areas, or is there not much of a difference?

For each of these questions, the response options were "easier," "not much of a difference," or "harder." For these questions, the indicated groups are African Americans, Latinos, low-income Americans, and Americans living in rural communities. All indicated groups are compared to a reference group that does in fact have an easier time accessing health care (white Americans, those who are better off financially, or those who live in urban areas).

Respondents in both the 2018 and 2020 surveys were also asked about their beliefs regarding the government's obligation to ensure access to health care.

> Do you agree or disagree with the following statement: It is the obligation of the government to ensure that everyone has access to health care as a fundamental right.

Respondents could answer on a five-point Likert scale, with 1 representing strongly agree and 5 representing strongly disagree.

Statistical Analysis

For each question answered on a Likert scale, we considered both the full distribution of responses and dichotomized responses, with somewhat agree and strongly agree set equal to 1, and neither agree nor disagree, somewhat disagree, and strongly disagree equal to 0. For questions on access, we also dichotomized responses. In the case of access to health care, each of the indicated groups in our questions do face greater difficulty accessing health care than the reference group; thus we distinguished between those who report a harder time versus those who say not much of a difference or an easier time. In some analyses for questions that were repeated, we also examine changes over time, creating indicator variables for any respondent who moved up (or down) the scale. While the full distribution of responses allows for greater variation and precision offered by a higher level of measurement, in our analysis we did not find that it led to meaningfully different results. Using the dichotomized responses allowed us to estimate linear probability models, which we present for ease of interpretation. In the appendix, we present both linear probability models and ordered logit models. Results were qualitatively similar.

We calculated unweighted and weighted descriptive statistics for our sample to assess whether there were any significant changes in the demographic characteristics of our sample over time and whether attrition in our sample could be predicted by demographic characteristics.

For the questions measured only in 2018, we examined the means of each of our key variables and made comparisons by race and ethnicity. Race and ethnicity were assessed in two separate questions, which we combined to create these mutually exclusive categories. We also conducted regression analysis to assess whether differences in opinions by race and ethnicity held after controlling for other characteristics. All regressions controlled for 2018 demographics: gender (male and female), age group (younger than 45, 45 to 64, and older than 65), education (less than high school, high school, some college, and college degree), family income (<$10,000, $10,000–$24,999, $25,000$–49,999, $50,000–$74,999, $75,000–$99,999, and $100,000 or more), marital status (married or living with a partner, separated, divorced, widowed, and single [never married]), and census region (East, Midwest, South, and West). All characteristics were categorical variables.

For variables that were assessed in both 2018 and 2020, we examined crosstabs of changes over time and two types of regression models. The first regressed a dichotomized response from 2020 on 2018 responses and demographics characteristics. The second examined who was most likely to change their responses. These regressions allow us to better understand what the characteristics are of people whose views are changing. If our dependent variables were continuous variables, these models would be akin to estimating a model in which the dependent variable was the change in the outcome. However, because we are interested in changes in a categorical variable, a simple difference does not suffice. First, a simple difference would result in many zeros, for people who expressed the same views in both periods, but people who said harder in both periods are likely very different from those who said easier in both periods. Second, many respondents are constrained and cannot move up (or down) the scale because they are already at the top (or bottom). To address this, we consider two groups of models with selected samples: those whose responses could move toward endorsing that some groups have more difficulty accessing care (i.e., those who did not respond harder in 2018), and those who could move down the scale toward reporting that some groups have an easier time accessing care (i.e., those who did not respond easier in 2018). As an example, in the models that assess who moves toward endorsing that African Americans have a harder time accessing health care than white Americans, we condition our sample on reporting easier or not much difference in 2018 and exclude those who report harder in 2018. Including those who already reported harder in 2018 would potentially bias our results, as these individuals are already at the top of the scale. They cannot report a higher level than harder in 2020. In the case of questions about access, these models can be thought of as measuring those who are not already endorsing the "truth," who moves toward the truth, and of those who are endorsing the truth (or equal access) who moves away from the truth. We exclude those who already endorse the truth, to better understand which individuals change their views and which do not. We consider similar models for the obligation of the government to provide access to care. All analysis was conducted in Stata 16.

Results

General Sociodemographic Characteristics

Table 2 provides descriptive statistics of the basic demographic characteristics of our sample. Columns 2 and 3 provide the unweighted characteristics, and columns 5 and 6 provide the weighted characteristics, both

Table 2 Demographic Characteristics of Sample

	Unweighted			Weighted	
	2018	2020	t-test (p)	2018	2020
Gender					
Male	43.8	43.8	0.00 (1.00)	48.1	48.1
Female	56.2	56.2	0.00 (1.00)	51.9	51.9
Race/ethnicity					
Non-Hispanic white	72.2	71.7	0.33 (0.74)	64.6	64.1
Non-Hispanic Black	9.2	9.2	0.00 (1.00)	11.7	11.7
Hispanic	13.4	13.4	0.00 (1.00)	18.0	18.0
Non-Hispanic Asian/PI	2.8	2.8	0.00 (1.00)	3.0	3.3
Non-Hispanic other	2.4	2.9	−0.92 (0.36)	2.6	3.0
Age group					
18–24	0.4	0.1	2.12 (0.03)	2.0	0.2
25–44	19.0	16.0	2.42 (0.02)	41.4	38.7
45–64	48.1	44.2	2.37 (0.02)	38.2	37.6
65+	32.5	39.7	−4.59 (0.00)	18.3	23.5
Education					
Less than high school	2.2	2.7	−0.96 (0.34)	5.5	6.9
High school	11.2	11.2	−0.05 (0.96)	29.9	30.1
Some college	34.6	33.7	0.62 (0.53)	28.2	25.8
College grad	52.0	52.4	−0.26 (0.79)	36.4	37.2
Family income					
<10k	4.4	3.7	1.01 (0.31)	7.5	6.1
10k–24,999	11.5	10.3	1.23 (0.22)	11.6	11.2
25k–49,999	22.8	23.8	−0.67 (0.50)	21.9	23.3
50k–74,999	22.4	21.1	0.94 (0.35)	24.6	20.3
75k–99,999	11.5	11.0	0.43 (0.66)	10.1	10.6
100k+	27.3	30.1	−1.82 (0.07)	24.3	28.5
Marital status					
Married or living with a partner	59.5	59.9	−0.23 (0.81)	60.4	61.6
Separated	2.2	2.2	0.00 (1.00)	3.7	2.4
Divorced	16.8	16.5	0.26 (0.79)	12.6	13.8
Widowed	6.2	6.8	−0.73 (0.46)	4.0	4.8
Single (never married)	15.4	14.7	0.55 (0.58)	19.3	17.5

weighted based on the sample characteristics in 2020. Column 4 displays t-tests comparing 2018 and 2020. For the most part, we see no significant changes in the characteristics of our sample. We also see that our sample ages during the two-year period, in part reflecting attrition and in part reflecting normal aging.

The Impact of COVID-19 on People of Color

Respondents were asked whether they agreed or disagreed that people of color faced more of a health and financial impact of COVID-19 than whites. In both cases, approximately 60% somewhat or strongly agreed, 27% to 30% neither agreed nor disagreed, and the remainder somewhat or strongly disagreed, as illustrated in figure 1.

We also examined differences by race and ethnicity and found that non-Hispanic Black respondents were significantly more likely to report that they strongly agreed with both statements than other racial groups (fig. 2). Of the non-Hispanic Black respondents, 58% reported that they strongly agreed that the pandemic has had a greater health impact on people of color, while for other races only 27% to 31% (p <0.01 for all comparisons). Of the non-Hispanic Black respondents, 59% reported that they strongly agreed that the pandemic has had a greater financial impact on people of color, while for other races only 25% to 34% (p <0.01 for all comparisons, except to non-Hispanic other races, where p = 0.027).

Table 3 presents selected results of a linear probability regression in which questions measuring the perceived health impact and financial impact on people of color are dichotomized. Columns 1 and 3 consider our base models. We find that non-Hispanic Black respondents are 16 percentage points more likely than non-Hispanic white respondents to somewhat or strongly agree that there is a greater health impact on people of color, and 31 percentage points more likely to agree that there is a greater financial impact. Hispanic respondents are seven percentage points more likely than non-Hispanic white respondents to agree that there is a stronger financial impact on people of color, but no more likely to endorse a difference in health impacts. Among non-Hispanic Asians, respondents are 19 percentage points less likely to agree there was a larger health impact than non-Hispanic whites, and those who report their race as Other were 13 percentage points more likely than non-Hispanic white respondents to somewhat or strongly agree that there was a greater financial impact.

We also find that both the views that there have been greater health and greater financial impacts on people of color are nine percentage points more likely to be endorsed by those in the highest income group ($100,000 or more) relative to those with income between $25,000 and $49,999. Both the views that there have been greater health and greater financial impact are 22 to 23 percentage points more likely to be endorsed by those with a college degree relative to those with a high school degree. We find that those living

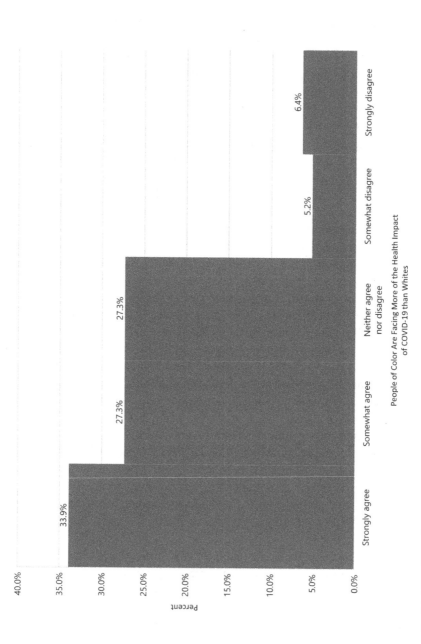

Figure 1 Distribution of responses to questions about impact of COVI9–19 on people of color.
Figure 1A Health impact.

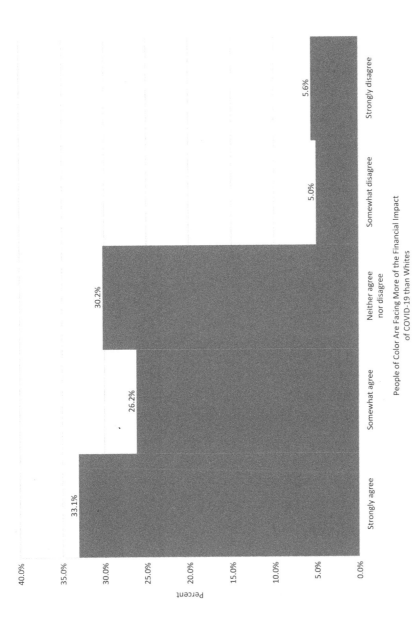

Figure 1B Financial impact.

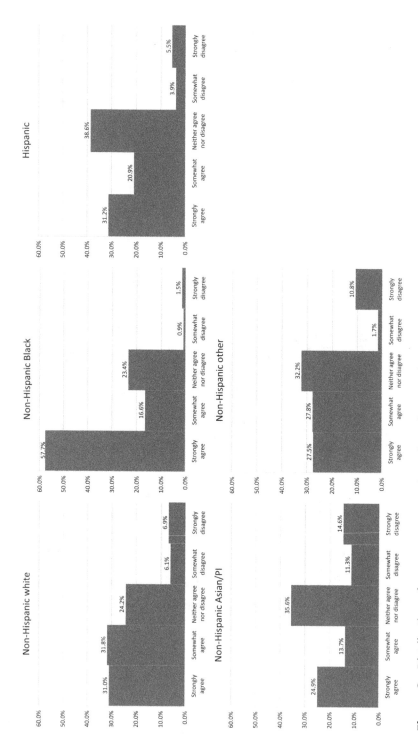

Figure 2 Distribution of responses to questions about impact of COVI9–19 on people of color by race and ethnicity.
Figure 2A Health impact.

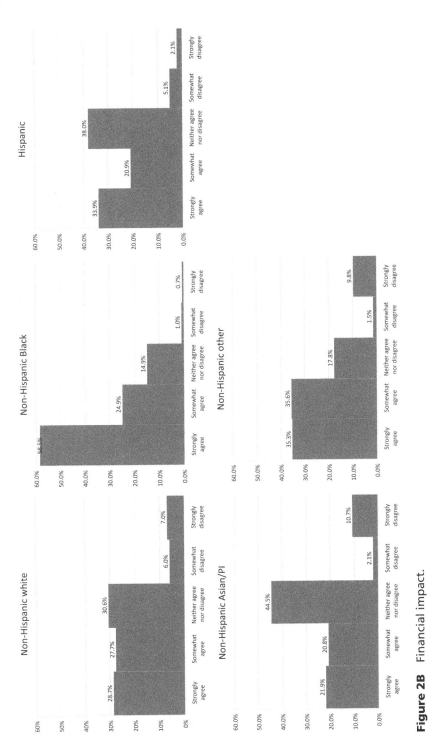

Figure 2B Financial impact.

Table 3 Selected Results of Linear Probability Model Predicting Somewhat or Strongly Agree COVID-19 Has Had a Greater Impact on People of Color

	More health impact on POC	More health impact on POC (additional controls)	More financial impact on POC	More financial impact on POC (additional controls)
Non-Hispanic Black (relative to non-Hispanic white)	0.162***	0.0565	0.312***	0.163***
	(0.0382)	(0.0369)	(0.0400)	(0.0369)
Hispanic (relative to non-Hispanic white)	−0.0418	−0.0931***	0.0721**	0.00494
	(0.0334)	(0.0318)	(0.0349)	(0.0318)
Non-Hispanic Asian/Pacific Islander (relative to non-Hispanic white)	−0.185***	−0.170***	−0.108	−0.0878
	(0.0647)	(0.0615)	(0.0676)	(0.0615)
Other non-Hispanic (relative to non-Hispanic white)	−0.00171	−0.0253	0.131**	0.0962*
	(0.0619)	(0.0584)	(0.0647)	(0.0584)
Female (relative to male)	0.0543**	0.0324	0.0295	0.00277
	(0.0215)	(0.0204)	(0.0225)	(0.0204)
Age 65 and older (relative to 44 and younger)	0.105***	0.0990***	0.0603*	0.0504
	(0.0334)	(0.0315)	(0.0349)	(0.0316)
Highest level of education: bachelors or higher (relative to high school)	0.222***	0.156***	0.226***	0.134***
	(0.0365)	(0.0348)	(0.0381)	(0.0348)
Family income $100,000 or higher (relative to $25,000 to $49,999)	0.0943***	0.0701**	0.0867**	0.0552*
	(0.0323)	(0.0306)	(0.0337)	(0.0306)

Table 3 (continued)

	More health impact on POC	More health impact on POC (additional controls)	More financial impact on POC	More financial impact on POC (additional controls)
South Census Region (relative to East)	−0.120***	−0.0828***	−0.103***	−0.0494*
	(0.0300)	(0.0284)	(0.0313)	(0.0284)
When African Americans need healthcare = not much of a difference		0.105**		0.145***
		(0.0470)		(0.0470)
When African Americans need healthcare = harder		0.222***		0.389***
		(0.0517)		(0.0517)
When Latinos need healthcare = harder		0.193***		0.185***
		(0.0466)		(0.0466)

Notes: Standard errors in parentheses. Variables in the regression included gender, age, education, income, marital status, and region. The complete regression models with all included controls are available in the online-only appendix.

*** p < 0.01, ** p < 0.05, * p < 0.1.

in the southern census region relative to the eastern census region are 12 and 10 percentage points less likely to endorse greater health and financial impacts, respectively. We also found that women (relative to men) and those older than 65 (relative to those younger than 45) are 5 and 11 percentage points, respectively, more likely to endorse a greater health impact.

In columns 2 and 4, we add controls for past views about whether African Americans and Latinos have a harder time accessing the health care (or "care") they need as measured in 2018. In columns 2 and 4, we see meaningful changes in the coefficients for non-Hispanic Black and Hispanic respondents compared to columns 1 and 3, suggesting, as we will see in the next section, that there is a high degree of collinearity between race and views about access to care for indicated groups in our questions about differences in access to health care. The signs and significance of other coefficients are more stable. We found that those who stated that it is harder for African Americans to access care were 22 percentage points more likely to indicate that the pandemic has had a greater impact on the health of people of color, and 39 percentage points more likely to indicate that it has had a greater financial impact, relative to those who said it was easier for African Americans to access care. Those who stated that it is harder for Latinos to access care were 19 percentage points more likely to indicate that the pandemic has had a greater health and financial impact on people of color, relative to those who said it was easier for Latinos to access care. We also found that those who stated that it is neither easier nor harder for African Americans to access care were 11 percentage points more likely to indicate that the pandemic has had a greater impact on the health of people of color and 15 percentage points more likely to indicate that it has had a greater financial impact, relative to those who said it was easier for African Americans to access care.

Views of Differences in Access

In both 2018 and 2020, respondents were asked about their views of differences in difficulty accessing health care for different groups. Panel data allows us to assess not only how the overall average has changed over time but also how many individuals have changed their views, which is important if there are groups that are moving in opposite directions. Table 4 presents crosstabs comparing results in 2018 and 2020 for each of the questions assessing differences in access for historically underserved groups, with each cell reporting a percentage of each 2018 response. For each indicated group, the majority of respondents reporting easier access moved away

Table 4   Differences in Perceptions in Access over Time
Table 4A When African Americans Need Health Care, Do You Think
It Is Easier or Harder for Them to Get the Care They Need
than It Is for White Americans?

	2018		
2020	Easier (7.4%)	Not much of a difference (52.6%)	Harder (40.0%)
Easier (4.1%)	23.5%	4.1%	0.6%
Not much of a difference (51.3%)	57.3%	72.4%	22.5%
Harder (44.6%)	19.2%	23.5%	76.9%
Total	100%	100%	100%

Table 4B   When Latinos Need Health Care, Do You Think
It Is Easier or Harder for Them to Get the Care They Need
than It Is for White Americans?

	2018		
2020	Easier (10.3%)	Not much of a difference (49.0%)	Harder (40.7%)
Easier (6.3%)	35.3%	4.5%	1.0%
Not much of a difference (49.8%)	53.4%	69.5%	25.2%
Harder (43.9%)	11.3%	25.9%	73.8%
Total	100%	100%	100%

Table 4C   When Low-Income Americans Need Health Care, Do You
Think It Is Easier or Harder for Them to Get the Care They Need
than It Is for Those Who Are Better Off Financially?

	2018		
2020	Easier (14.6%)	Not much of a difference (19.0%)	Harder (66.4%)
Easier (8.6%)	26.3%	8.2%	4.7%
Not much of a difference (26.2%)	37.6%	52.5%	16.1%
Harder (65.3%)	36.1%	39.2%	79.2%
Total	100%	100%	100%

Table 4D When Americans Living in Rural Communities Need Health Care, Do You Think It Is Easier or Harder for Them to Get the Care They Need than It Is for Those Who Live in Urban Areas?

	2018		
2020	Easier (4.2%)	Not much of a difference (34.3%)	Harder (61.5%)
Easier (2.9%)	13.2%	3.5%	1.8%
Not much of a difference (36.9%)	62.9%	62.5%	20.8%
Harder (60.3%)	23.9%	34.0%	77.4%
Total	100%	100%	100%

from that perception. Of respondents who reported easier access for African Americans in 2018, 77% reported not much difference or harder in 2020, and 65% of those reporting easier access for Latinos in 2018 reported not much difference or harder in 2020. Of those reporting easier access for low-income Americans in 2018, 74% reported not much difference or harder in 2020, and 87% of those reporting easier access for Americans living in rural communities in 2018 reported not much difference or harder in 2020. The percentage of 2018 reports of harder access for these groups moving away from that perception toward easier ranged from 21% to 26%.

Table 5 presents the selected results of linear probability regression models that predict if 2020 respondents endorsed that each group had a harder time accessing health care, controlling for their response to the same question in 2018 and for demographic characteristics. In all cases, those who reported harder in 2018 were significantly more likely to report harder again in 2020 (reflecting the stability observed in table 4), and those who reported not much difference for African Americans and Latinos in 2018 were more likely to report that it was harder in 2020 for those groups than those who reported easier in 2018. Controlling for 2018 responses, non-Hispanic Black respondents were more likely than non-Hispanic white respondents to report that African Americans and low-income Americans have a harder time accessing care. Hispanic respondents were less likely than non-Hispanic white respondents to report that Latinos, low-income Americans, and those living in rural areas have a harder time accessing care. Those in the middle age group (45 to 64) were generally less likely than those in the youngest age group to report that access was harder for our indicated groups, while those in the highest income and education

Table 5 Selected Results of Linear Probability Model Predicting That Getting Health Care Is Harder for Indicated Underserved Groups When They Need Care

	African Americans relative to white Americans	Latinos relative to white Americans	Low-income relative to high-income Americans	Americans in rural relative to urban areas
Responses in 2018				
When African Americans need healthcare = not much of a difference	0.0756** (0.0380)			
When African Americans need healthcare = harder	0.607*** (0.0391)			
When Latinos need healthcare = not much of a difference		0.135*** (0.0336)		
When Latinos need healthcare = harder		0.667*** (0.0346)		
When low-income Americans need healthcare = Harder			0.417*** (0.0292)	
When Americans in rural communities need healthcare = Harder				0.362*** (0.0577)

(continued)

Table 5 Selected Results of Linear Probability Model Predicting That Getting Health Care Is Harder for Indicated Underserved Groups When They Need Care (*continued*)

	African Americans relative to white Americans	Latinos relative to white Americans	Low-income relative to high-income Americans	Americans in rural relative to urban areas
Demographics				
Non-Hispanic Black (relative to	0.0904**	0.0302	0.0796**	−0.0123
non-Hispanic white)	(0.0353)	(0.0350)	(0.0360)	(0.0364)
Hispanic (relative to	−0.0411	−0.0656**	−0.112***	−0.0383
non-Hispanic white)	(0.0304)	(0.0304)	(0.0315)	(0.0318)
Female (relative to male)	0.0513***	0.0420**	0.0130	0.0393*
	(0.0195)	(0.0194)	(0.0203)	(0.0204)
Age 45–64 (relative to 44	−0.0968***	−0.0888***	−0.0905***	−0.00599
and younger)	(0.0282)	(0.0281)	(0.0292)	(0.0295)
Highest level of education:	0.140***	0.160***	0.134***	0.186***
bachelors or higher	(0.0334)	(0.0332)	(0.0344)	(0.0351)
(relative to high school)				
Family income $50,000 or higher	0.0122	0.0106	0.0442	0.0558*
(relative to $25,000 to $49,999)	(0.0293)	(0.0292)	(0.0304)	(0.0307)
Observations	1,841	1,840	1,843	1,843
R-squared	0.371	0.377	0.214	0.204

Notes: Standard errors in parentheses. Variables in the regression included gender, age, education, income, marital status, and region. The complete regression models with all included controls are available in the online-only appendix.

*** p<0.01, ** p<0.05, * p<0.1.

groups and women were generally more likely to report that access was harder for our indicated groups.

Table 6 shows selected results for models that investigate respondents who move toward endorsing that indicated groups have a harder time getting the care they need and those respondents who move away from endorsing that indicated groups have a harder time getting the care they need. Among those who did not recognize inequities in access in 2018, very few variables are correlated with moving toward reporting that it is harder for our indicated groups to access health care. Among those that had not previously reported harder, non-Hispanic Black respondents are more likely to move toward harder access for African Americans. Among those that had not previously reported easier, Hispanic respondents are more likely to move toward easier for all indicated groups. Higher income and higher education are positively associated with moving toward reporting harder, and negatively associated with moving toward reporting easier, while lower-income respondents are more likely to move toward easier. Non-Hispanic white, lower-income, or less-educated respondents who previously did not recognize inequities were less likely to change their views than non-Hispanic Black, higher income, or more highly educated respondents. In all models, we find that those whose views were previously at the extreme are more likely to shift their views than those whose views were in the middle.

Beliefs about the Government's Obligation to Ensure Access to Health Care

In both 2018 and 2020, respondents were asked whether they agree that it is an obligation of the government to ensure access to health care as a fundamental right. We can again assess how many individuals have changed their opinions, which is important if there are groups that are moving in opposite directions. Table 7 presents a crosstab comparing results in 2018 and 2020. Nearly 14 percentage points more individuals report that they strongly agreed in 2018 compared to 2020. About half of the respondents strongly disagreeing in 2018 reported strongly or somewhat agreeing in 2020. We see that same proportion of opinion shifting among those somewhat disagreeing in 2018. Among those strongly agreeing in 2018, 12% moved to somewhat or strongly disagreeing in 2020. Of those neither agreeing nor disagreeing in 2018, 43% somewhat or strongly agreed in 2020, and 14% somewhat or strongly disagreed in 2020.

Table 6 Selected Results of Linear Probability Model Predicting Changes in Endorsement That Getting Care Is Harder for Indicated Underserved Groups

	Move toward harder				Move toward easier			
	African Americans relative to white Americans	Latinos relative to white Americans	Low-income relative to high-income Americans	Americans in rural relative to urban areas	African Americans relative to white Americans	Latinos relative to white Americans	Low-income relative to high-income Americans	Americans in rural relative to urban areas
When African Americans need healthcare = not much of a difference	−0.468*** (0.0412)							
When African Americans need healthcare = harder					0.146*** (0.0151)			
When Latinos need healthcare = not much of a difference		−0.376*** (0.0380)						
When Latinos need healthcare = harder						0.143*** (0.0153)		
When low-income Americans need healthcare = not much of a difference			−0.257*** (0.0430)					

Table 6 (continued)

	Move toward harder				Move toward easier			
	African Americans relative to white Americans	Latinos relative to white Americans	Low-income relative to high-income Americans	Americans in rural relative to urban areas	African Americans relative to white Americans	Latinos relative to white Americans	Low-income relative to high-income Americans	Americans in rural relative to urban areas
When low-income Americans need healthcare = harder							0.118*** (0.0245)	
When Americans in rural communities need healthcare = not much of a difference				−0.421*** (0.0686)				
When Americans in rural communities need healthcare = harder								0.178*** (0.0183)
Non-Hispanic Black (relative to non-Hispanic white)	0.199*** (0.0661)	0.0701 (0.0663)	0.147 (0.0895)	0.0188 (0.0636)	−0.0338 (0.0267)	0.0270 (0.0277)	−0.0503 (0.0340)	0.0705** (0.0305)
Hispanic (relative to non-Hispanic white)	0.0558 (0.0435)	0.0352 (0.0461)	0.0414 (0.0660)	0.0549 (0.0603)	0.0675*** (0.0235)	0.0729*** (0.0239)	0.115*** (0.0301)	0.0795*** (0.0264)

(continued)

Table 6 Selected Results of Linear Probability Model Predicting Changes in Endorsement That Getting Care Is Harder for Indicated Underserved Groups (continued)

	Move toward harder				Move toward easier			
	African Americans relative to white Americans	Latinos relative to white Americans	Low-income relative to high-income Americans	Americans in rural relative to urban areas	African Americans relative to white Americans	Latinos relative to white Americans	Low-income relative to high-income Americans	Americans in rural relative to urban areas
Highest level of education: bachelors or higher (relative to high school)	0.0960** (0.0440)	0.0723 (0.0463)	0.0568 (0.0683)	0.121** (0.0617)	−0.0451* (0.0262)	−0.117*** (0.0272)	−0.131*** (0.0335)	−0.108*** (0.0290)
Family income $100,000 or higher (relative to $25,000 to $49,999)	0.108*** (0.0418)	0.110** (0.0436)	0.0486 (0.0662)	0.142** (0.0616)	−0.0517** (0.0225)	−0.0131 (0.0233)	−0.0220 (0.0292)	−0.0478* (0.0253)
Observations	1,066	1,047	533	591	1,714	1,670	1,593	1,784
R-squared	0.150	0.110	0.115	0.116	0.092	0.098	0.082	0.077
Excludes	Harder in 2018	Harder in 2018	Harder in 2018	Harder in 2018	Easier in 2018	Easier in 2018	Easier in 2018	Easier in 2018

Notes: Standard errors in parentheses. Variables in the regression included gender, age, education, income, marital status, and region. The complete regression models with all included controls are available in the online-only appendix.

*** $p < 0.01$, ** $p < 0.05$, * $p < 0.1$.

Table 7   Differences in Attitudes of Government Obligations over Time

	2018				
2020	Strongly agree (31.8%)	Somewhat agree (21.1%)	Neither agree nor disagree (15.8%)	Somewhat disagree (12.1%)	Strongly disagree (19.3%)
Strongly agree (45.8%)	80.6%	36.6%	21.0%	15.7%	37.6%
Somewhat agree (22.4%)	10.1%	41.6%	21.7%	35.7%	13.7%
Neither agree nor disagree (15.0%)	7.1%	10.1%	43.2%	18.0%	8.2%
Somewhat disagree (8.5%)	0.8%	5.3%	11.5%	20.8%	14.2%
Strongly disagree (8.4%)	1.4%	6.4%	2.5%	9.7%	26.3%
Total	100%	100%	100%	100%	100%

The first column of table 8 presents a linear probability regression model (similar to table 5) that predicts whether in 2020 respondents reported somewhat or strongly agree that it is the government's obligation to ensure access to health care, controlling for their response to the same question in 2018 and for demographic characteristics. The second and third columns are similar to table 6, reporting those who move toward or away from strongly agree. Those who reported somewhat or strongly agree in 2018 were significantly more likely to report somewhat or strongly agree again in 2020. Non-Hispanic Black and Hispanic respondents (compared to non-Hispanic white respondents) and women (compared to men) were more likely to agree in 2020 (controlling for 2018 responses) and more likely to move toward agreement that government has an obligation to ensure access to health care. Those with the highest levels of education are more likely to somewhat or strongly agree, and less likely to move away from strongly agreeing. We also found strong regional differences, with those in the eastern census region mostly likely to agree and to move toward agreement.

Discussion

Our analysis suggests that approximately 60% of respondents believed that people of color faced more of a health and financial impact of COVID-19 than whites, which is broadly consistent with earlier findings by Sarah E. Gollust and colleagues (2020) and from the Kaiser Family Foundation

Table 8 Selected Results of Linear Probability Model Predicting That Somewhat or Strongly Agree It Is the Obligation of the Government to Ensure Access to Health Care

	Somewhat or strongly agree	Move toward strongly agree	Move away from strongly agree
Government obligation = strongly agree, 2018	0.414*** (0.0266)		0.0353 (0.0298)
Government obligation = somewhat agree, 2018	0.280*** (0.0293)	−0.347*** (0.0342)	0.0812** (0.0317)
Government obligation = neither agree nor disagree, 2018	−0.0334 (0.0346)	−0.262*** (0.0405)	0.0452 (0.0361)
Government obligation = domewhat disagree, 2018	−0.0619* (0.0338)	−0.101** (0.0393)	
Non-Hispanic Black (relative to non-Hispanic white)	0.145*** (0.0354)	0.199*** (0.0568)	−0.0508 (0.0366)
Hispanic (relative to non-Hispanic white)	0.120*** (0.0307)	0.149*** (0.0429)	−0.0749** (0.0324)
Female (relative to male)	0.0404** (0.0199)	0.0593** (0.0281)	−0.0149 (0.0211)
Highest level of education: bachelors or higher (relative to high school)	0.0678** (0.0338)	−0.0209 (0.0469)	−0.0606* (0.0353)
Midwest Census Region (relative to East)	−0.107*** (0.0320)	−0.133*** (0.0466)	0.0328 (0.0334)
South Census Region (relative to East)	−0.150*** (0.0276)	−0.149*** (0.0403)	0.0933*** (0.0292)
West Census Region (relative to East)	−0.121*** (0.0286)	−0.170*** (0.0421)	0.0444 (0.0301)
Observations	1,843	1,233	1,447
R-squared	0.239	0.131	0.029

Notes: Standard errors in parentheses. Variables in the regression included gender, age, education, income, marital status, and region. The complete regression models with all included controls are available in the online-only appendix.

*** $p < 0.01$, ** $p < 0.05$, * $p < 0.1$. .

(Hamel et al. 2020). The results presented here also suggest that there are significant racial and ethnic differences in views regarding the impact of the COVID-19 pandemic on minorities, and that there are also differences in how individuals' views have changed in the time between 2018 and 2020. Our panel data allows us to observe changes across the same individuals from a period well before the pandemic began to the summer of 2020.

Of particular note, while the pandemic has impacted both African Americans and Latinos more negatively than white Americans, we observe dramatic differences in responses to several questions for these groups. While non-Hispanic Black respondents were much more likely than non-Hispanic white respondents to note that people of color had been more negatively impacted by the pandemic (both in terms of health and financial impacts), Hispanic respondents' reports were more similar to non-Hispanic whites. These findings are broadly consistent with previous work suggesting that whites are less likely to perceive racial inequities (Kraus, Rucker, and Richeson 2017; Kraus and Tan 2015; Richeson and Nussbaum 2004). However, our findings contrast with surveys administered in spring 2020 by Gollust and colleagues (2020) that found no differences between Blacks and whites in perceptions of racial differences in the health impacts of COVID-19, suggesting that racial differences in COVID-19 impact may have become more salient to non-Hispanic Blacks since the early days of the pandemic.

Our findings do not provide information that allows us to tease out what specific mechanisms might be at work here (e.g., differences in social networks, motivated cognition related to a commitment to a race-neutral ideology, etc.). Nor do they speak directly to why there are differences among specific nonwhite groups. However, our results also show that those respondents (controlling for race and ethnicity) who in 2018 endorsed greater difficulties for designated groups in accessing care were more likely to report that the pandemic has had a greater impact on people of color. This finding suggests that those who are most likely to endorse the idea that the pandemic has had disproportionate impacts on people of color are those who were already aware of inequities in our society. Thus our analysis appears broadly consistent with the idea that beliefs about racial inequity change either slowly, or only in response to deep shocks to the system (Scheidel 2018). Furthermore, it may take more than news coverage of inequities to change the minds of some groups. It is impossible to separate the effects of the pandemic from the effects of the greater attention to racial inequity brought on by the killings of George Floyd and Breonna Taylor and subsequent protests; however, our results suggest that those groups who were most likely to change were the same groups that were already most likely to report awareness of inequities.

Indeed, when respondents are asked about difficulties accessing health care, we find that more respondents report there are differences related to income and rural or urban location than race, and that the stark inequities highlighted by the pandemic only slightly changed these perceptions. In fact, in 2020 Hispanic respondents were less likely than non-Hispanic white respondents to report that Latinos had a harder time accessing health care than white Americans and more likely to move toward reporting that Latinos have an easier time accessing care. Non-Hispanic Black respondents, on the other hand, were more likely in the midst of the pandemic to recognize inequities and move toward recognizing inequities. There were two key groups that were likely to report inequities and to move toward recognizing inequities: those whose incomes were more than $100,000 and those with a college education or more. The pandemic, resulting inequities, and civil unrest around the country related to racial inequities appear to have had very unequal impacts on views of inequity.

We saw striking changes in the share of respondents reporting that it is the obligation of the government to ensure access to health care, with nearly 14 percentage points more individuals reporting that they strongly agreed this was an obligation of the government than in 2018, and a total of 68% of respondents in 2020 somewhat or strongly agreeing this was an obligation. This increase appears to be appreciably larger than earlier increases in support for a government role in health noted at the beginning of the article (Kiley 2018). These increases were most strong among non-Hispanic Black and Hispanic respondents, women, those with higher education, and those living in the eastern census region. This result for Hispanics is particularly interesting, since they were also less likely in 2020 than in 2018 to report that Latinos have a harder time accessing health care. It is interesting that the views of inequity in access to care are not necessarily tied to views about government's obligation to ensure access to health care, even though the government could play a central role in reducing inequity by ensuring that everyone has access to care.

Conclusion

The events of 2020 (pandemic, recession, and racial tension and civil unrest) have disproportionately affected historically marginalized racial and ethnic groups in our society and have brought heightened attention to these inequities. This could be an opportunity to educate the public about inequities that are common in our society and encourage more social policies to help address these inequities. However, our results contribute to the growing evidence of polarization in our society and that many views remain stable. Even in the face of evidence in the news media on a near daily basis, views of equity changed only slightly. Deeper research is needed to understand why those who do not report inequities continue to stick to their views, and a more concerted effort to help people under-stand the experiences of other groups may be needed. In particular, among the less-educated, lower-income, and white groups, views of equity were less likely to change.

While there have been only small changes in perceptions of inequity, there have been larger changes in the perception that the government has an obligation to ensure access to care, a key tool in addressing inequity. This suggests that the increase in the demand for government ensuring access to health care is not driven by an increased concern about inequity but rather by other changing views.

There are several important limitations of our work that speak to the need for further research. First, there are other potential explanations that are unmeasured. The unwillingness to report racial and ethnic inequity may stem from a desire to appear race neutral (Richeson and Nussbaum 2004); we see no similar unwillingness to report inequity based on income or rural locations. Our 2018 survey contains no other measures of views about race. Similarly, other measures of political ideology and affiliation are not included in our survey. Second, our 2020 survey was fielded primarily in early July. At that time, the COVID-19 pandemic had significantly impacted large cities, and the second wave of cases seen in the summer primarily in the southern and rural areas was only just beginning. As COVID-19 infections spread across the country, views may continue to evolve. In future surveys, including one in the field at the time of writing, one to be fielded in January, and another to be fielded in early spring, we may see attitudes continue to shift, awareness grow or wane. Third, we are not able to measure the views and perspectives of American Indians/Native populations in our research, as they make up too small a share of our sample to separately report results for this group. However, given the profound impact of the pandemic on Native populations, this is an important limitation of our research.

Even in the face of a deadly pandemic, one that has killed dispropor-tionately more African Americans and Latinos, many in our society do not recognize that there are inequities in access to health care and disparate health and financial impacts of the pandemic on these groups. While some groups are changing their views, changing these deeply seated views to more accurately reflect reality will continue to be a challenge. While there have been changes, it remains to be seen whether these changes will be persistent as the pandemic continues. There seems to be growing support for the government ensuring access to health care; however, other policies to address inequity may require further shifts in public opinion. Shifting perspectives is a key part of how societies make changes and progress.

Large-scale events, such as the COVID-19 pandemic and the resulting recession and attention to inequity, have in the past provided opportunities for change. We will continue to follow these respondents to see if changes in attitudes endure over time or dissipate.

■ ■ ■

Katherine Carman is a senior economist and director of the Center for Financial and Economic Decision Making at the RAND Corporation. Her research focuses on how information and perceptions affect individual behavior and decisions. She is particularly interested in the ways that knowledge and trust can influence views, values, and mindset. Her work spans several topic areas, including financial decisions, health behaviors, voting behavior, political attitudes, and labor decisions. She has developed surveys and new data to shed new light on these important questions. Previously she was a professor at Tilburg University in the Netherlands and a research scholar at Harvard University.
kcarman@rand.org

Anita Chandra is the vice president and director of RAND Social and Economic Well-Being and a senior policy researcher at the RAND Corporation. The division also manages RAND's Center to Advance Racial Equity Policy. She leads studies on civic well-being and urban planning; community resilience and long-term disaster recovery; public health emergency preparedness; effects of military deployment; equity, health in all policies, and advancing a culture of health; and child health and development. Throughout her career, she has engaged governmental and nongovernmental partners to consider cross-sector solutions for improving community well-being and to build more robust systems, implementation, and evaluation capacity.

Carolyn Miller is a senior program officer with the Research-Evaluation-Learning unit at the Robert Wood Johnson Foundation. Prior to joining the foundation in 2013, she was a research consultant, conducting quantitative and qualitative research for commercial and academic research organizations, foundations, nonprofit organizations, and professional associations. She has held research positions with Mathematica Policy Research, the Gallup Organization, and Princeton Survey Research Associates.

Christopher Nelson is a senior political scientist at the RAND Corporation and a professor of policy analysis at the Pardee RAND Graduate School. He has more than 25 years of experience as a policy analyst. Primarily he works on health systems and preparedness, but he has also worked on public safety, transportation, energy, and education. Previously he served on the faculty of Carnegie Mellon University and held research staff positions at Western Michigan University and the Illinois General Assembly.

Jhacova Williams is an associate economist at the RAND Corporation. She is an applied microeconomist focusing primarily on economic history and cultural economics. Her previous work has examined Southern culture and the extent to which historical events have impacted the political behavior and economic outcomes of Southern Blacks. Recent examples include historical lynchings and the political participation of Blacks and Confederate symbols and labor market differentials. She has also done a series of projects investigating the role of structural racism in shaping racial economic disparities in labor markets.

Acknowledgments

The authors thank Delia Bugliari and Linnea Warren May for research assistance. This research was funded by the Robert Wood Johnson Foundation (award no. 74430). The funding body offered input on the study design and interpretation of data, but ultimately the RAND study team had final determination of all research design, analysis, and interpretation choices. The manuscript was written by the RAND study team.

References

Aknin, Lara B., Christopher P. Barrington-Leigh, Elizabeth W. Dunn, John F. Helliwell, Justine Burns, Robert Biswas-Diener, Imelda Kemeza, et al. 2013. "Prosocial Spending and Well-Being: Cross-Cultural Evidence for a Psychological Universal." *Journal of Personality and Social Psychology* 104, no. 4: 635–52.

Artiga, Samantha, and Kendal Orgera. 2019. "Key Facts on Health and Health Care by Race and Ethnicity." Kaiser Family Foundation, November 12. www.kff.org/report -section/key-facts-on-health-and-health-care-by-race-and-ethnicity-coverage-access -to-and-use-of-care/.

Braveman, Paula, Elaine Arkin, Tracy Orleans, Dwayne Proctor, and Alonzo Plough. 2017. *What Is Health Equity? And What Difference Does a Definition Make?* Princeton, NJ: Robert Wood Johnson Foundation.

Burstein, Paul. 2003. "The Impact of Public Opinion on Public Policy: A Review and an Agenda." *Political Research Quarterly* 56, no. 1: 29–40.

Bye, Larry, Alyssa Ghirardelli, and Angela Fontes. 2016. "American Health Values Survey." Robert Wood Johnson Foundation, June 30. www.rwjf.org/en/library /research/2016/06/american-health-values-survey-topline-report.html.

Carman, Katherine Grace, Anita Chandra, Delia Bugliari, Christopher Nelson, and Carolyn Miller. 2020. "COVID-19 and the Experiences of Populations at Greater Risk Description and Top-Line Summary Data—Wave 1, Summer 2020." www .rand.org/t/RRA764-1 (accessed April 22, 2021).

Carman, Katherine Grace, Anita Chandra, Carolyn Miller, Matthew Trujillo, Douglas Yeung, Sarah Weilant, Christine DeMartini, Maria Orlando Edelen, Wenjing Huang, and Joie D. Acosta. 2016. "Development of the Robert Wood Johnson Foundation National Survey of Health Attitudes: Description and Top-Line Summary Data." www.rand.org/pubs/research_reports/RR1391.html (accessed April 22, 2021).

Carman, Katherine Grace, Anita Chandra, Sarah Weilant, Carolyn Miller, and Margaret Tait. 2019. "2018 National Survey of Health Attitudes: Description and Top-Line Summary Data." www.rand.org/pubs/research_reports/RR2876.html (accessed April 22, 2021).

CDC (Centers for Disease Control and Prevention). 2020. "COVID-19 Hospitalization and Death by Race/Ethnicity." August 18. www.cdc.gov/coronavirus/2019-ncov/covid-data/investigations-discovery/hospitalization-death-by-race-ethnicity.html.

Chandra, Anita, Joie Acosta, Katherine Carman, Tamara Dubowitz, Laura C. Leviton, Laurie Martin, Carolyn E. Miller, et al. 2016. "Building a National Culture of Health: Background, Action Framework, Measures and Next Steps." www.rand.org/pubs/research_reports/RR1199.html (accessed April 22, 2021).

Citrin, Jack. 1979. "Do People Want Something for Nothing: Public Opinion on Taxes and Government Spending." *National Tax Journal* 32, no. 2: 113–29.

Conover, Pamela Johnston, and Stanley Feldman. 1984. "Group Identification, Values, and the Nature of Political Beliefs." *American Politics Quarterly* 12, no. 2: 151–75.

Diepeveen, Stephanie, Tom Ling, Marc Suhrcke, Martin Roland, and Theresa M. Marteau. 2013. "Public Acceptability of Government Intervention to Change Health-Related Behaviours: A Systematic Review and Narrative Synthesis." *BMC Public Health* 13, no. 1: 756.

Gollust, Sarah E., and Joseph N. Cappella. 2014. "Understanding Public Resistance to Messages about Health Disparities." *Journal of Health Communication* 19, no. 4: 493–510. doi.org/10.1080/10810730.2013.821561.

Gollust, Sarah E., and Julia Lynch. 2011. "Who Deserves Health Care? The Effects of Causal Attributions and Group Cues on Public Attitudes about Responsibility for Health Care Costs." *Journal of Health Politics, Policy and Law* 36, no. 6: 1061–95. doi.org/10.1215/03616878-1460578.

Gollust, Sarah E., Rachel I. Vogel, Alexander Rothman, Marco Yzer, Erika Franklin Fowler, and Rebekah H. Nagler. 2020. "Americans' Perceptions of Disparities in Covid-19 Mortality: Results from a Nationally-Representative Survey." *Preventive Medicine* 141: 106278.

Goren, Paul, Christopher M. Federico, and Miki Caul Kittilson. 2009. "Source Cues, Partisan Identities, and Political Value Expression." *American Journal of Political Science* 53, no. 4: 805–20.

Hamel, Liz, Audrey Kearney, Ashley Kirzinger, Lunna Lopes, Cailey Muñana, and Mollyann Brodie. 2020. "KFF Health Tracking Poll—June 2020." Kaiser Family Foundation, June 26. www.kff.org/racial-equity-and-health-policy/report/kff-health-tracking-poll-june-2020/.

Hessami, Zohal. 2010. "The Size and Composition of Government Spending in Europe and Its Impact on Well-Being." *Kyklos* 63, no. 3: 346–82.

Hook, Cayce J., and Hazel Rose Markus. 2020. "Health in the United States: Are Appeals to Choice and Personal Responsibility Making Americans Sick?" *Perspectives on Psychological Science* 15, no. 3: 643–64.

IOM (Institute of Medicine). 2003. *Unequal Treatment: Confronting Racial and Ethnic Disparities in Health Care.* Washington, DC: National Academies Press.

Jacobs, Lawrence. 1992. "Institutions and Culture: Health Policy and Public Opinion in the US and Britain." *World Politics* 44, no. 2: 179–209.

Kiley, Jocelyn. 2018. "Most Continue to Say Ensuring Health Care Coverage Is Government's Responsibility." Pew Research Center, October 3. www.pewresearch .org/fact-tank/2018/10/03/most-continue-to-say-ensuring-health-care-coverage-is -governments-responsibility/.

Kraus, Michael W., Julian M. Rucker, and Jennifer A. Richeson. 2017. "Americans Misperceive Racial Economic Equality." *PNAS* 114, no. 39: 10324–31.

Kraus, Michael W., and Jacinth J. X. Tan. 2015. "Americans Overestimate Social Class Mobility." *Journal of Experimental Social Psychology* 58: 101–11.

Krosnick, Jon A., and Donald R. Kinder. 1990. "Altering the Foundations of Support for the President through Priming." *American Political Science Review* 84, no. 2: 497–512.

Markus, Gregory B. 2001. "American Individualism Reconsidered." In *Citizens and Politics,* edited by James H. Kuklinski, 401–31. Cambridge: Cambridge University Press.

Nellis, Ashley. 2016. "The Color of Justice: Racial and Ethnic Disparity in State Prisons." Washington, DC: Sentencing Project.

Oishi, Shigehiro, Ulrich Schimmack, and Ed Diener. 2011. "Progressive Taxation and the Subjective Well-Being of Nations." *Psychological Science* 23, no. 1: 86–92.

Pacheco, Julianna, and Elizabeth Maltby. 2017. "The Role of Public Opinion—Does It Influence the Diffusion of ACA Decisions?" *Journal of Health Politics, Policy and Law* 42, no. 2: 309–40. doi.org/10.1215/03616878-3766737.

Pagel, Christina, David W. Bates, Don Goldmann, and Christopher F. Koller. 2017. "A Way Forward for Bipartisan Health Reform? Democrat and Republican State Legislator Priorities for the Goals of Health Policy." *American Journal of Public Health* 107, no. 10: 1601–3.

Perrin, Andrew. 2020. "23% of Users in US Say Social Media Led Them to Change Views on an Issue; Some Cite Black Lives Matter." Pew Research Center, October 15. www.pewresearch.org/fact-tank/2020/10/15/23-of-users-in-us-say-social-media -led-them-to-change-views-on-issue-some-cite-black-lives-matter/.

Pollard, Michael, and Matthew D. Baird. 2017. "The RAND American Life Panel: Technical Description." August 24. www.rand.org/pubs/research_reports/RR1651 .html.

Richeson, Jennifer A., and Richard J. Nussbaum. 2004. "The Impact of Multiculturalism versus Color-Blindness on Racial Bias." *Journal of Experimental Social Psychology* 40, no. 3: 417–23.

Salter, Phia S., Glenn Adams, and Michael J. Perez. 2018. "Racism in the Structure of Everyday Worlds: A Cultural-Psychological Perspective." *Current Directions in Psychological Science* 27, no. 3: 150–55.

Scheidel, William. 2018. *The Great Leveler: Violence and the History of Inequality from the Stone Age to the Twenty-First Century.* Princeton, NJ: Princeton University Press.

Shedd, Carla. 2015. *Unequal City: Race, Schools, and Perceptions of Injustice*. New York: Russell Sage Foundation.

Swidler, Ann. 1986. "Culture in Action: Symbols and Strategies." *American Sociological Review* 51, no. 2: 273–86.

Thomas, Deja, and Juliana Menasce Horowitz. 2020. "Support for Black Lives Matter Has Decreased since June but Remains Strong among Black Americans." Pew Research Center, September 16. www.pewresearch.org/fact-tank/2020/09/16/support-for-black-lives-matter-has-decreased-since-june-but-remains-strong-among-black-americans/.

US Census Bureau. 2019. "Selected Characteristics of Health Insurance Coverage in the United States." data.census.gov/cedsci/table?q=s2701&t=Health%20Insurance&y=2019&tid=ACSST1Y2019.S2701 (accessed April 26, 2021).

Wilson, Valerie. 2020. "Racial Disparities in Income and Poverty Remain Largely Unchanged amid Strong Income Growth in 2019." Economic Policy Institute, *Working Economics Blog*, September 16. www.epi.org/blog/racial-disparities-in-income-and-poverty-remain-largely-unchanged-amid-strong-income-growth-in-2019/.

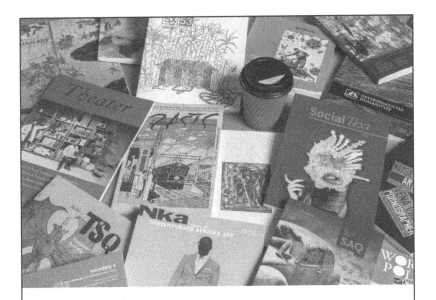

Keep up to date on new scholarship

Issue alerts are a great way to stay current on all the cutting-edge scholarship from your favorite Duke University Press journals. This free service delivers tables of contents directly to your inbox, informing you of the latest groundbreaking work as soon as it is published.

To sign up for issue alerts:

1. Visit **dukeu.press/register** and register for an account. You do not need to provide a customer number.

2. After registering, visit **dukeu.press/alerts**.

3. Go to "Latest Issue Alerts" and click on "Add Alerts."

4. Select as many publications as you would like from the pop-up window and click "Add Alerts."

read.dukeupress.edu/journals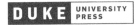

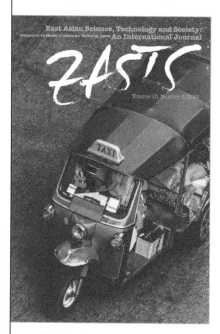
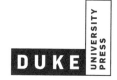